THE SOUL DIET

Panfili's Quantic Orthomolecular Biohacking Approach to Body Mind & Spirit

Written By

ADOLFO PANFILI

Hardcover: 978-1-967828-86-9

Paperback: 978-1-967828-75-3

Published by:
Pine Book Writing
www.PineBookWriting.com
R-10225 Yonge St Suite #250, Richmond Hill, ON L4C 3B2, Canada.

Printed in the United States of America

Films That Will Make You Proud To Be Human

Movies are undeniably one of the most powerful therapeutic tools ever created. The narratives, rooted in the hero myth, draw on ancient mythological models that are present in every cultural tradition across the globe. No civilization exists without its myths.

Within each of you, there's a hero waiting to be awakened, eager to embark on the alchemical journey of transformation, to embody the richest archetypes worthy of Pirandello's brilliant *One, No One, One Hundred Thousand…* The Cowboy, the Flawless Knight, the Warrior, the Martyr, the Guardian Angel, the Seeker, the Lover, the Destroyer, the Ruler, the Magician, the Sage, the Fool, the Outlaw—these characters are like the tarot cards in a cosmic pantomime, playing pivotal roles in our personal battles or standing as the dolls in our stories.

Much like chemical catalysts, heroes create change without changing themselves. Unstoppable, they face the most impossible odds, risking everything at every turn—think Bruce Willis in his action-packed glory.

Life needs heroes, and heroes need life—specifically, the lives of others with whom they interact in ways that reality can't fully contain. Just as every Boy Scout needs the classic "good deed" to complete their day, so does the hero need challenges to shape their journey.

The hero shines with their own light, so bright that anyone who orbits them reflects this glow. Their radiance catalyzes evolution in those around them. They penetrate our collective myths, emerging as figures who are timeless, ageless, steadfast like an ancient oak tree. Whether arriving on horseback or in a spaceship, the mythical hero will always return—fearless and untarnished, like a rock, to seek out the next battle or quest to face, much like the legendary Hercules and his never-ending Labors.

A woman, a family—they are often insufficient to deter the hero from their ultimate sacrifice, propelling them into a life that's disconnected from the ordinary world. With few human traits, they easily betray reality, seeking temporary but deeply therapeutic escapes for a rebirth, often in the span of just under two hours of cinematic bliss.

Enter the Mentor. Like Pallas Athena in the *Odyssey*, the Mentor brings wisdom and guidance, helping to recharge the faded batteries of our hero. Think of John Rambo, who, after retreating to a monastery in Cambodia, is called back to action by the enthusiasm of his Colonel.

Mentors are emissaries of the divine, veiled angels, delivering the wisdom of the gods in small, potent doses. They represent the higher self, the divine spark within each of us, capable of making us the heroes of our childhood dreams. Thanks to them, our heroes, once dormant, now sparkle once again in our hearts—hearts that may have felt deflated by lives that seem as irrelevant as an old, discarded rubber band. Characters like Jiminy Cricket, Geppetto, the Blue-Haired Fairy, or Sean Connery in *Highlander* symbolize the highest aspirations of our inner heroes.

Mentors embody the ideal version of what the hero hopes to become. Many heroes, in fact, are simply seeking mentors because their parents have not been the guiding figures they needed.

Every doctor, every therapist is, in their own way, a mentor—redeeming the hero that's always been slumbering in your heart, waiting to be awakened. Perhaps you don't need a cappuccino for that wake-up call, just a bucket of popcorn and a Coke.

Enjoy the movie, and enjoy your recovery!

Here are some films that are universally recognized for their ability to make you exclaim: "Gosh, I'm just happy to be alive!"

Great movies offer a deeply fulfilling experience, leaving you with a sense of satisfaction that can cleanse your emotions. Whether you're crying, laughing, or both, the catharsis they provide serves as a natural remedy for anyone looking to shake off the weight of heavy emotions. Instead of popping pills to calm your racing heart, grab a ticket for a soul-nourishing film or rent one of the recommended classics.

These films adhere to the essential pedagogical canons that inspire positivity and help reconcile you with humanity. For centuries, viewers have been captivated by the timeless struggle between good and evil, with good ultimately triumphing—perhaps after a few grueling twists and turns. Watching these films leaves you with the comforting knowledge that, despite the trials of life, there's always something valuable to learn about human nature.

And you can enjoy these emotional journeys without worrying about gratuitous or disturbing violence often found in films that lack substance. It's a solid antidepressant therapy at a reasonable price and without any of the unpleasant side effects. Sometimes, seeing truly is believing!

The Classic Hero's Journey

1. Star Wars Saga (1977–present) – The quintessential hero's journey with Luke Skywalker, the Jedi, and the battle between light and dark.

2. The Lord of the Rings Trilogy (2001–2003) – Frodo, Aragorn, and Gandalf embody different heroic archetypes on an epic journey.
3. The Matrix (1999) – Neo's path from an ordinary hacker to "The One" follows mythological transformation.
4. Gladiator (2000) – Maximus as the Warrior, Martyr, and Ruler in a quest for justice.
5. Braveheart (1995) – William Wallace as the rebellious warrior and martyr for freedom.

The Unbreakable Warrior

6. Die Hard Series (1988–2013) – Bruce Willis' John McClane is the perfect inoxidizable hero.
7. Mad Max: Fury Road (2015) – Max and Furiosa fight against tyranny in a dystopian wasteland.
8. The Dark Knight Trilogy (2005–2012) – Batman as the Ruler, Warrior, and Seeker of justice.
9. John Wick Series (2014–present) – The relentless warrior archetype in modern noir.
10. The Revenant (2015) – Hugh Glass as the ultimate survivor and avenger.

The Mythic and the Mystical

11. Inception (2010) – The Seeker and the Magician in a journey through the subconscious.

12. The Green Knight (2021) – A knight's quest for honor, steeped in myth and legend.
13. The Fountain (2006) – A journey through love, time, and transformation.
14. Doctor Strange (2016) – The Magician archetype unlocking cosmic secrets.
15. Pan's Labyrinth (2006) – A dark fairy tale about courage and metamorphosis.

The Outlaw and the Trickster

16. Joker (2019) – The Fool and the Criminal archetypes in a psychological descent.
17. The Wolf of Wall Street (2013) – The Ruler turned Trickster in a capitalist playground.
18. No Country for Old Men (2007) – A brutal meditation on fate and chaos.
19. The Good, the Bad and the Ugly (1966) – Cowboys as mythic figures in the Wild West.
20. Scarface (1983) – The rise and fall of a criminal anti-hero.

The Spiritual and the Visionary

21. The Last Samurai (2003) – The Seeker finding meaning in the Samurai way.
22. Cloud Atlas (2012) – Interwoven destinies of souls seeking enlightenment.

23. Dune (2021) – Paul Atreides as the reluctant hero navigating fate.
24. The Tree of Life (2011) – A poetic exploration of existence.
25. The Truman Show (1998) – A man breaking free from illusion to seek truth.

These are movies as an uplifting, cathartic experience! There are also films that can make you exclaim, "Gosh, guys, I'm just happy to be alive!"—films that leave you with a renewed faith in life, people, and the magic of storytelling.

Movies That Restore Your Faith in Humanity

1. It's a Wonderful Life (1946) – A timeless classic about the value of life and human connections.
2. Forrest Gump (1994) – A journey through history with innocence, love, and perseverance.
3. The Pursuit of Happyness (2006) – Overcoming hardship with sheer determination and love.
4. Life Is Beautiful (1997) – Finding joy and hope even in the darkest times.
5. The Green Mile (1999) – A deeply human story of kindness and miracles.

Feel-Good Comedies & Romances

6. Amélie (2001) – The power of small acts of kindness and whimsy.
7. Love Actually (2003) – A heartwarming tapestry of love in all its forms.
8. Groundhog Day (1993) – A cynical man's transformation into his best self.
9. Little Miss Sunshine (2006) – A dysfunctional family's journey toward joy.
10. Julie & Julia (2009) – Cooking, passion, and finding purpose.

Uplifting Adventures & Stories of Triumph

11. Dead Poets Society (1989) – Seizing the day and embracing self-expression.
12. The Intouchables (2011) – A moving and humorous tale of friendship across social divides.
13. The Secret Life of Walter Mitty (2013) – A stunning ode to adventure and breaking free.
14. Slumdog Millionaire (2008) – Destiny, love, and resilience in the face of adversity.
15. Billy Elliot (2000) – Chasing dreams against all odds.

Animated Films That Warm the Soul

16. Up (2009) – An unforgettable journey about love, loss, and rediscovery.
17. Inside Out (2015) – A beautiful look at emotions and growing up.
18. Coco (2017) – A moving story of family, music, and memory.
19. Finding Nemo (2003) – An inspiring adventure about perseverance and love.
20. WALL-E (2008) – A hopeful vision of love and humanity's potential.

Musicals & Pure Joy on Screen

21. La La Land (2016) – Dreams, love, and the bittersweet beauty of life.
22. Mamma Mia! (2008) – A blast of joy set to ABBA's greatest hits.
23. The Greatest Showman (2017) – A celebration of individuality and spectacle.
24. Singin' in the Rain (1952) – A classic that radiates happiness.
25. Bohemian Rhapsody (2018) – A triumphant ode to music and self-acceptance.

These films offer that much-needed emotional reset, reminding us why life is worth embracing, even in its messy, unpredictable beauty.

Table Of Contents

Introduction:
Hope Is Born From Every Truth

The first healing comes from hope
this is kept in everyone's soul,
woe to him who deprives another human being of this wealth.

As soon as I graduated in medicine, I was convinced that diseases were formidable adversaries, sacred monsters to be battled with sword drawn and spear in hand—like an indomitable knight of Arthurian legend.

The challenge of single combat with illness seemed both obvious and inevitable for a doctor who had chosen to share in the suffering of his fellow human beings—whether in the solemn halls of a hospital ward or the intense, almost sacred heat of an operating theater. Perhaps, beneath it all, there was an unspoken and misguided aspiration: the hope that, by confronting suffering so closely, one might somehow become immune to death, pain, and the turmoil they bring.

Yet, as the years passed, the once-unshakable convictions I held began to falter under the weight of clinical experience. Reality, unfiltered and uncompromising, revealed to me the stark relativity of my role in the grand scheme of cosmic and individual well-being.

Watching patients fall ill, endure pain, recover, or succumb—unable to alter the relentless course of fate—was one of the first cold showers that chilled my soul. Observing how some individuals with the same diagnosis triumphed while others lost the ultimate battle forced me to acknowledge the presence of another silent yet no less significant force in human existence: hope.

Hope, in its highest form, is faith—the fundamental fuel of all healing. But faith is not merely a passive or abstract belief; it is the driving force behind our capacity to act, to engage our will, and to make decisive choices. It is not an intellectual construct detached from reality but the very essence of excellence in any endeavor, including the journey toward healing.

For many of the patients I encountered, the fear of losing was far stronger than the desire to overcome their illness.

I am profoundly grateful to all those who, through their suffering and humanity, have taught me that healing is an alchemy—a transformation that occurs through multiple pathways of the human soul. Faith, like a laser beam, can pierce through any obstacle, embodying the power of irrepressible, unstoppable love—

an indispensable catalyst for unlocking the hidden, miraculous potential within every human being.

After more than twenty years in medicine, I have come to understand—sometimes at my own expense—that patients are souls inhabiting bodies, not the other way around. Healing begins with the soul, which proclaims its restoration before the body echoes it in atoms, cells, organs, and systems—supported, but never dictated, by the work of a physician. We are merely assistants to what the great father of medicine, Hippocrates, called *Vis Medicatrix Naturae*—the healing force of nature.

You and the world around you are not static matter, but a continuous act of creation—a fluid expression of being, forever in motion. Disease, in this light, is not merely a malfunction of the body but a disruption in the divine flow that silently, yet powerfully, pulses within each of us. It is a hidden cry for help from a heart in distress.

Both the celestial and the earthly realms belong to you—if only you dare to believe in your path and seek what you have long feared to find.

The purpose of my life, is to rediscover the lost thread of Ariadne within each heart. To help you find your way home, to reconnect with the beautiful soul within you, waiting to be heard.

You always have the power to change, to shape, to transform your destiny for the better. Never settle for limitations. Always search for that glimmer of light leading to growth. Only those who have the courage to believe in their true selves will reclaim their inner paradise. This book, and the authors behind it, are dedicated to this very mission.

Your decision to purchase this book was a wise one. However, statistics suggest that only ten percent of readers ever make it beyond the first chapter. Our hope is that you defy this disheartening prediction.

Wherever life has taken you, the time has come to demand more from yourself. Do not let the knowledge and insights within these pages go to waste. Read them, reread them, and with each pass, you will discover something new—an ever-deepening source of wisdom and inspiration.

Though this book spans only about two hundred pages, within these lines, you may find the very answers you have been waiting for. So do not stop. Keep reading.

This book is dedicated to these aspirations and to all those who have made them a guiding light—for themselves and for others.

February 1600

"And he said that he died a martyr and willingly,
and what would his ascended soul be like without it
with that smoke in Heaven"

Giordano Bruno's last words before the execution on
Thursday 17 February 1600.

The soul's time machine is free to wander across worlds, stars, and galaxies. Now, the hand of the centuries seems to halt nearly four hundred years ago: February 1600.

On that freezing February morning, the wind lashed mercilessly against the curtains of the houses, while a light rain barely softened the chill left behind by the night. The Jubilee of 1600, proclaimed by Pope Clement VIII, illuminated the streets with the glow of pilgrims swarming into the Holy City, seeking indulgences.

Like a courtesan adorned for a grand occasion, Baroque Rome—mother, sister, daughter, and lover all at once—was preparing to welcome more than three million foreigners expected for the Holy Year, embracing them in its raw and sordid splendor.

Yet, at that very hour, the slow, creaking wheels of a mule-drawn cart rattled over the cobblestones, making its way from the Tor di Nona prison. It carried no joyous tidings. Amidst the icy gusts of the northern wind, flashes of blue and turquoise flickered defiantly across Campo de' Fiori, where a spectacle was about to unfold.

That Thursday morning was a day of celebration, for at last, that wicked Dominican friar from Nola—a most obstinate heretic—was to be burned alive. His blasphemy against the Blessed Virgin and all the saints had earned him a fate far worse than the twelve years of imprisonment imposed by the Holy Office. The dogmas he had trampled were sacred and indisputable. No mercy for the wicked; forgiveness was reserved only for the jubilant pilgrims rejoicing in the twelfth Jubilee of the new century.

The former friar, tormented in both body and mind by endless hours of torture, his flesh ravaged by years of disgraceful captivity, swayed like an empty reed in the wind as the macabre procession dragged him forward. Yet, even as fever and festering wounds consumed his frail body, his spirit soared—untamed and unbroken. His mind, his soul, and his thoughts had not been enslaved by the ferocious inquisitors, who had in vain sought to extinguish his deepest aspirations.

Like Prometheus, he had dared to steal the sacred fire of the gods, wresting it from the Sun's dominion. A son of both sun and earth, a citizen of the world and the universe, he was a wanderer trapped in a body soon to be returned to its divine creator—like a horse finally led back to its celestial stable.

Anathema upon him! He had tried to profane the Sacred Fire, from which all arts are born, offering its secrets to ordinary mortals and thereby undermining the power of sanctioned knowledge. Science, he had claimed, was a paradox: while it freed a select few predestined spirits, it enslaved the ignorant and the fearful—those triumphant beasts who reigned over a world darkened by their own shadows. Science, to him, was a circle within a circle, a never-ending loop.

This time, like Zeus himself, the prelates would deliver a punishment far worse than mere chains. They would bind him to the stake, and rather than an eagle devouring his immortal liver, they would summon fire to purge his outcast soul—the soul of the Magician of Nola.

No Hercules would come to his rescue. No hero would strike down the Holy Office's vulture with a single, merciful arrow. There would be no redemption, no reprieve. The Holy Father demanded a severe example to be made of this defiant man who had sought martyrdom on his own terms, indifferent to bodily torment, proclaiming with impunity that his soul would rise with the smoke of his pyre, uniting with the great soul of the Universe.

The cursed Dominican friar from Nola—this obstinate heretic—had not been tamed by red-hot pincers, nor by the cruel rack. His impenitence had been confirmed *ipso iure* by an avalanche of dubious and wavering testimonies—no fewer than thirty in total. Among them, an eyewitness named Scioppio would later recall at least fourteen.

- Denying transubstantiation.
- Questioning the virginity of Mary.
- Having sojourned in heretical lands and lived in the guise of a heretic.
- Having authored *The Expulsion of the Triumphant Beast* against the Pope.
- Asserting the existence of innumerable and eternal worlds.
- Proclaiming reincarnation and the possibility that a single sacrilegious soul may inhabit two or more bodies.
- Declaring magic to be good and lawful.
- Identifying the Holy Spirit with the soul of the world.
- Claiming that Moses feigned his miracles and invented the Law.
- Declaring that Holy Scripture is nothing more than a dream.

- Believing that even demons shall be saved.
- Holding the opinion that Pre-Adamites existed.
- Asserting that Christ is neither God nor divine but a deceiver and a magician.
- Declaring that the prophets and apostles were also magicians, and that almost all met grim fates.

Reading through these spurious accusations, one can't help but imagine that a modern sixth-grader, especially one hooked on *Stranger Things*, would be just as liable—if not more so—than the poor friar himself, tried for heresy and witchcraft.

The priceless legacy Giordano Bruno offered us—sealed with the holocaust of his own life—is a blazing metaphor of man's ability to break free from the obsessive fear of death. He placed the eagle of hope into the hands of humanity, gifting them with fire—the primal force from which all things arise and draw their strength, just as *Prometheus Bound* tells us (vv. 7, 110, 250).

The myth that Bruno reinterprets is embedded in the very etymology of the name *Prometheus*, which means "forethought"—a testament to the subtle and penetrating rebellion of the spirit striving to reclaim the divine spark of intelligence from which it originates.

Throughout history, both collective and individual identities have anchored themselves to dominant influences, solidifying ancient behavioral patterns to avoid awakening the unsettling specter of change. While the Middle Ages exalted the spirit at the expense of the mind, in 1478, the Spanish monarchs Ferdinand of Aragon and Isabella of Castile sought Pope Sixtus IV's authorization to appoint inquisitors in their kingdoms. Their intent was ostensibly to safeguard against the growing presence of ethnic minorities—comprising 100,000 Jews and 300,000 Muslims—amidst a total population of fewer than six million.

The Spanish Inquisition, much like the *Sant'Uffizio* in Rome, ostensibly aimed to protect the ruling class. However, in reality, it served as a ruthless mechanism to preserve the status quo of an entrenched religious hierarchy. It also functioned as a barrier against scientific inquiry—often the only means of social advancement available to these marginalized groups, whose intellectual and demographic growth threatened the established ecclesiastical order.

With its irrepressible and pervasive force, independent thought projected an unsettling, ascending energy into the highest echelons of the religious world, exposing a deep-seated malaise within the fabric of Christian doctrine. Originally conceived in the spirit of Christic love, this doctrine had been shipwrecked by bureaucratic manipulations that distorted its superhuman ideal—often at the hands of ministers who ascended to the papal throne through nepotism and iconoclastic ambition rather than spiritual merit.

The human aspiration for intellectual freedom—unshackled from the sectarian and religious obscurantism of pseudo-culture—demanded the expansion of real human potential, limitless in its divine origin. This quest for enlightenment survived only through the alchemy of the spirit, the awakening of consciousness, and even through the transcendence of suffering. Pain, in this context, became a launching pad for the soul, enabling it to break free from the confines of the body and rediscover its true, unified self. The annihilation of the ego thus became a path to redemption.

The Church of the time saw Jewish, Islamic, and freethinking influences—such as those of Bruno—as an existential threat to its monopoly on power, a force capable of undermining the corporate stronghold of what was, in essence, the greatest multinational institution of the era: the Roman Catholic Church. Yet the seed of transformation had already taken root in the stony ground of an emerging unitary and absolute state, where religious unity was increasingly viewed as a crucial pillar of survival. Those who challenged this unity—including Bruno—were deemed a menace to the rural aristocracy, which jealously guarded its incense-scented privileges.

As the flames of Lutheran anti-papal polemics spread, Italy—once the unrivaled cultural epicenter of the world—began to lose its preeminence. From that point onward, Catholicism became synonymous with backwardness and obscurantism, rendering Erasmus of Rotterdam's famous dictum—*"Italians, we are all noble and cultured"*—obsolete and anachronistic.

What, then, can be said of the inquisition led by Cardinal Archbishop of Milan, Saint Charles Borromeo, who condemned the entire Benedictine congregation of Monte Cassino as heretical—merely for daring to adopt a critical stance against the feudal Roman Church? Christ had preached a radically different morality, yet his message had been twisted and deformed by the dark forces of power. The defiance of those pure souls who resisted tyranny and preached enlightenment—only to be sacrificed on the altar of knowledge—was, in many ways, inevitable in the long night of the Renaissance.

How many more Giordano Brunos must be immolated on the altar of human dignity? How many more crimes against freedom and respect will be carried out under the auspices of self-righteous institutions?

Morality is elastic and ever-changing—an expensive private luxury, especially for the religious institution of the Roman Catholic Church. Only now, after centuries, has it humbly bowed its head, sprinkling itself with ashes in an act of penance for the misdeeds committed in its name—misdeeds perpetrated under the false pretense of safeguarding a Christ who, like Bruno and many others, chose to die for an idea.

No, these deaths have not been in vain. They continue to serve those who remain—those who know how to read between the lines—with an unthinkable strength and the relentless drive to ensure that truth prevails. And yet, how many more Giordano Brunos must be burned alive? How many more Jesus Christs must wither upon the arms of a cross before Truth can finally emerge, sovereign and unchallenged?

Truth does not belong to a fixed moment—it is the daughter of every instant, especially of those in which it feels most unwelcome. Truth cannot truly exist until the last human being has lived their experience and spoken their word.

Thank you, Bruno, for the healing you have instilled in our hearts—for restoring to us the most precious gift of all: Hope.

Change The Body By Changing The Mind

"Imagination is more important than knowledge and rules the world"
Albert Einstein.

Statistical studies indicate that approximately seventy percent of learning in the first six years of life shapes the ability to acquire new information. This phase is also the most fertile in terms of imagination.

A strong imagination is therefore essential for learning quickly and effectively. We should dedicate more time and respect to nurturing creative imagination in school education, stimulating and developing it as much as possible into adulthood—and perhaps even beyond.

When have you ever heard a parent say, "I'm worried because my child has an incredible imagination!" or "That child always has his head in the clouds..."? Instead, many seem to believe that a child's imagination is valuable only insofar as it entertains and amuses adults.

A vivid imagination is as valuable as a strong memory and serves as the foundation of any solid education, as well as a strategy for solving most existential dilemmas.

People like Einstein and Edison possessed extraordinary imaginations. Albert Einstein, in particular, reached his scientific conclusions about space-time by mentally projecting himself into a virtual extra-planetary world, where he could roam freely, riding on pale moonbeams. His ability to regress into childhood-like imaginative thinking helped him become one of the greatest intellectuals of all time.

Aging itself is not the worst affliction; rather, it is the loss of visual and imaginative power.

Some individuals recover more quickly than others from serious illnesses and surgical procedures, simply following the administration of a placebo (from the Latin meaning "to give relief"), an inert substance with no pharmacological properties. Yet, in certain individuals with heightened imaginative capacity, it can psychologically support and accelerate healing. Conversely, the same substance can also trigger negative effects, known as the nocebo effect, where patients experience serious and unpleasant side effects. In both cases, it is the expectation tied to the given molecule that makes the critical difference and explains the ambivalent outcomes.

Among the substances with placebo-nocebo effects, we must certainly include words, diagnoses (whether given or withheld), and the attitude of a doctor, surgeon, or any other authoritative figure toward the patient.

Telling a sick person outright, "You have only six months to live because you have cancer," is an act of unnecessary sabotage to their immune and defense strategies—not to mention a cynical and inhumane approach. Why not instead tell them that, in addition to the mortality associated with the disease, there are also cases of people who, though facing immense difficulty, manage to fight and achieve recovery? Their behaviors deserve study and emulation.

Over four thousand confirmed cases of recovery have been analyzed by the Institute of Noetic Sciences in San Francisco (Sausalito), California, as part of the Neoplastic Remission Project. This information is readily available online, particularly for those skeptical about the possibility of recovering from cancer.

According to Siegel, at least 90% of people who recover from cancer undergo a significant change in their quality of life before achieving remission.

Accepting that an emotional event can trigger the onset of cancer is as controversial as Columbus believing the Earth was round when everyone thought it was flat. This is why many prefer to claim an initial diagnostic error when an "unexpected" recovery changes the narrative, rather than admitting the possible link between mind, body, and soul.

Hamer, the author of the theory that bears his name, had to defend his thesis before the medical association to which he belonged, presenting numerous cases of patients who recovered from the "disease of the century" without drugs, simply by resolving the underlying emotional conflict.

This perspective does not seek to trivialize or minimize such an intense and dramatic issue. Rather, it aims to understand the strategies at its root (see chapter on cancer).

Older individuals often report memory decline. Many of them have let their imagination deteriorate to the point that their minds are no longer capable of generating images that adhere to the firmament of their thoughts.

For a therapist, the supreme imaginative act was once to invoke a spirit or deity to catalyze the healing process. Many unrepentant sorcerers and witches were burned at the stake simply for being slow to align with the emerging medical trends of their time. This practice of exorcism eventually became obsolete when the discovery of vitamins led to the eradication of scourges like scurvy, beriberi, pellagra, and rickets.

In 1922, the discovery of insulin by three Canadian researchers from Toronto—Frederick Banting, Charles H. Best, and John J.R. Macleod—gave an immense boost to clinical pharmacology, allowing diabetic individuals to live with a quality and duration of life previously unthinkable.

The apotheosis of this medical revolution came in 1929 with Sir Alexander Fleming's synthesis of penicillin at St. Mary's Hospital in London. This discovery dramatically altered the course of medicine, ushering in an era that would revolutionize public health.

Devastating illnesses like pneumonia and bronchopneumonia could be tamed overnight. Patients who had been feverish and near death one day were back on their feet the next. Like all experimental drugs, penicillin—the "panacea for all infections"—was initially extremely expensive. In fact, hospitals resorted to boiling the urine of treated patients to extract and administer the antibiotic to others, ensuring equally rapid recoveries at a cost manageable for the healthcare systems of the time.

The mystery of health and healing has always fascinated humanity, which, since ancient times, has considered it the result of invisible and intangible forces, requiring appeasement through rituals and offerings to capricious deities.

For centuries, diseases and epidemics were interpreted as manifestations of divine wrath. The healer stood alone against these fearful and enigmatic forces, much like a modern-day Indiana Jones venturing into the depths of the psyche to access the encrypted language of the soul. In this entronautical journey, an individual's willpower meant little, beyond invoking the mercy of a supreme and solitary God, nestled deep within the recesses of the true self.

With the advent of fundamental drugs—vitamins, insulin, and penicillin—medical science began producing cures at a rate reminiscent of an assembly line, much like the automobile industry. This had nothing to do with faith, which, as a counterbalance, was increasingly relegated to the fringes of the relentless pursuit of health at all costs.

In some circles, even suggesting a connection between faith and healing was considered offensive, particularly in cases where the rigid mechanisms of post-Newtonian science demanded practicality and tangible results.

Separating body and soul was almost a palliative necessity for some therapists who wanted to shake off the ancient and obsolete exorcistic legacies of folk medicine—often practiced by charlatans and impostors more concerned with the "health" of their wallets than that of their unfortunate patients.

Human beings have always fallen ill and recovered, and at least once in their lifetime, unfortunately... they die, even without pharmaceutical intervention. This suggests that medicine should not be considered an irreplaceable pillar in the evolution of human civilization.

Leonardo painted the Mona Lisa without ever taking an aspirin for the headaches that plagued him during his creative immersions. Michelangelo sculpted the Pietà and adorned the Sistine Chapel without ingesting painkillers to relieve the cervicobrachialgia (neck pain extending to the upper limbs) that tormented him. Julius Caesar, who suffered from epilepsy, did not die because he lacked diphenylhydantoin, just as Jesus and his disciples wandered fearlessly through Palestine without ever having been vaccinated.

The Path Of Joint Scales: The Way Of The Right Means

"When you have fully understood there is nothing to understand"

KoanZen.

It is therefore legitimate to assume that even exorcistic, magical, and religious medicines contain their share of truth, without suggesting that the reader should distrust so-called official medicine—the very foundation upon which humanity relies to rediscover the Ariadne's thread of total well-being.

Medicine is both an art and a science. Let this noble institution, intended by God to save mankind, also draw from real and undeniable socio-economic and cultural contexts, which should not be ignored by the scientific community, even if they are often wrapped in mystical, metaphysical, and verbose choreographies.

Anything that promotes healing while respecting the ethical and biological laws of nature has the right to stand at the bedside of the sick, without restrictions of caste, ideology, or convenience.

The Path of the Joint Scales, corresponding to the Buddha's Way of the Golden Mean, particularly refers to the line of clear alchemical inspiration that guided the Medicine Man—the ancestor of today's Homo Medicus. The principle of "solve et coagula," understood as the arrhythmic interplay of dissolutions and condensations, becomes in Panfhealing® the methodical regularity of practices based alternatively on Graduated Wisdom or on Powers that are as effective and concrete as they are non-ordinary.

In the oscillation between techniques, beyond the external chaos, lies a subtle, empty harmony—estranged from ordinary thought, fundamentally occult—which suggests to the modern therapist a personal path toward the transhuman.

Many great and mysterious diseases, upon whose cold cliffs the hopes of allopathic healers of all ages have shattered, have melted like snowflakes in the sun before the presence of the great healers of humanity. Figures like Hippocrates, Asclepius, Avicenna, and Theophrastus Bombastus, known as Paracelsus, pursued a transformative approach to medicine, often finding their most complete justification in miracles—phenomena that overturn the classical understanding of the known physical world.

In this context, the Fire of Imagination merging into the Water of Panta Rei ("everything flows") becomes a force capable of shaping reality—creating and regenerating life from the decay of disease, resurrecting it from death, thereby reenacting Genesis, the original creation of the world from nothingness. Vision transforms into the tangible reality of the Fantastic Universe. The final symbol of reunification is the Phoenix, the mythical bird that lives, dies, and regenerates from its ashes—a metaphor for the Cosmic Hermaphrodite, the entity that both creates and is created, endlessly regenerating from the Gnostic Abyss of Nothingness, much like the Ouroboros serpent of Hindu mythology.

Based on these considerations, it is possible to reclaim the concept of total healing as a holistic process arising from the perfect synergy of soul, mind, and body—coining the neologism: "Panfhealing® ."

In Greek, "Pan" means "all," while in English, "Healing" and "Feeling" respectively mean recovery and perception (any reference to the names of the authors is not purely coincidental, ed.).

Rediscover your emotions, as they may be the silent tenants of symptoms and illnesses—the protagonists of the grand "commedia dell'arte" of life. Recognize pain as the greatest ally in regaining and maintaining health.

If all diseases stem from a separation from the archetypal model of the ideal life we were meant to live, then the path to individual healing lies in rediscovering this inner and unifying Ariadne's thread, from which the alchemy of total well-being flows like clear spring water—henceforth synonymous with orthomolecular healing.

Soto Zen And Rinzai Zen: Getting Sick To Understand

Woe to that nation which passes from religion to conviction, from the country path to the city avenue, from wisdom to logic. Woe to that nation that does not weave what it wears, does not plant what it eats, does not press the grapes whose juice it drinks.

Woe to that submissive nation that looks at the ostentation of the victor as a mirror of virtue, the nation in whose eyes the turpitude of the ruler is beauty. Woe to that nation that fights injustice in dream, but surrenders to evil in waking hours.

Woe to that nation that raises its voice only at funerals, Showing consideration only beside graves and waiting to rebel until a sword blade hangs around her neck.

Woe to that nation whose politics is abstruseness, whose philosophy is deceit, whose industry is recycling. Woe to that nation that acclaims the ruler with the roll of the drums, and then drives him away with whistles and greets the new master with songs and trumpet sounds.

Woe to that nation where the wise man is speechless, the champion does not see, the lawyer is a stutterer. Woe to that nation where every tribe claims to be a nation.

Kahlil Gibran - Spiritual Saying

However, everything is not always as easy as it seems and things do not go as smoothly as one would like, in fact, orthomolecular healing passes through the gauntlet of awareness, which can only be pursued after having faced the most evocative, fascinating, but often frightening of journeys, the one through your inner self. Getting sick to understand each other, or rather to better understand the world, the cosmos, the universe, etc. An illness is often an excellent opportunity to feel more loved and pampered, as happens to your child who concocts a non-existent fever in the morning because you are neglecting him, for example. Do many of you suffer from depression because you have an unsatisfying personal relationship, which makes you unhappy, yet continue the ooze of this exhausting relationship? Why never? Often out of laziness, because you waited for a change (almost always from the other) without even lifting a finger. The old adage: "he who leaves the old road for the new one ... knows what he leaves, but does not know what he finds" is certainly suitable for you, because despite being unhappy, you have been overwhelmed by fear of the unknown, suffering for you well harsher and scarier than living with the partner of your nightmares. On the other hand, if you are in the mood for proverbs, isn't it perhaps "better an egg today than.. a chicken tomorrow?". Well! Why not instead expect a nice hen today, in spite of the cheeky wisdom of proverbs and who wrote them? Try it! Those who don't have the courage to dare don't get, this seems to be Murphy's iron Law, which smiles on the brave. Happy people have had the courage to do what their heart prompted them, largely ignoring the specters of change and now they draw the right tributes. Fear and laziness push human beings into the abyss of sloth, where not even the great poet Dante manages to find the right to a suitable place in his hell, leaving them to grope helpless outside the scorching environments. Don't hope for the AAA (American Automobile Association) help of a charming prince or a fairy with blue hair and start to... lift your butt! As in recovering a dusty bicycle abandoned in a dark cellar since childhood, it will be necessary to take courage in both hands, arm oneself with time and begin the descent into the underworld of the deepest individual innate: rediscovering the true City of the Soul, the real factory of feelings and emotions, with exceptional therapists themselves... The evolutionary path of most men, on the other hand, is based on the Water element, and implies a gradual, mental, pragmatic initiation carried out in ordinariness and possibly under the guidance of a master. This is a slow and demanding work, like the load loaded on the back of a powerful but placid bovine, certainly less dangerous, since it is structured on a controlled progression of the delivery of the teachings By analogy this path could be analogous to Soto Zen, which in Eastern Zen practice is defined as: "The Path of Gradual Enlightenment", otherwise known to Western alchemists as the Wet Path. This category of limiting thoughts prevents people from changing, at least until they reach the limit of extreme pain tolerance, they explode by shaking off the previous fear of the unknown in an adrenaline-pumping acidifying flash and end the relationship with the wrong person or rather they say enough to extra kilos, because tuxedo pants or a Valentino suit no longer fit. It is only a matter of time! Gioberti considered in his divine model the fusion of time and space as an absolute intuition in the context of infinity, while by definition human time is finite, but not for those who decide to truly heal. The extreme experience, the straw that overflows the fateful vase is like Archimedes' lever and can literally lift monstrous weights of behavioral styles that otherwise you would not have been able to move even a millimeter. A woman during an earthquake that occurred many years ago in Irpinia, Italy, had lost her little son under the rubble of her collapsed house. Desperate and weeping, her mother did not accept to leave the place of the catastrophe, continuing to call her child by name, who had been missing for many hours under the cement, between bricks and rubble. Suddenly faint and distant screams invoking the magical name mom began to reach her baby ear. Happy and dismayed at the same time by the good news of the child still alive and by the emerging need to get him out of that trap of tons of stones as soon as possible, she began her greatest adventure with time and with God. She began to dig like a madwoman with her hands alone, and meanwhile the cries of the child grew closer and more desperate, as the pebbles were gradually removed from the young girl's hands, which were covered more and more with wounds and blood. The baby of a few months of life was dying suffocated by that mountain of rubble. In the meantime, some soldiers from the rescue group rushed to help her speed up that desperate operation, but they finally had to stop in front of a last chestnut lintel weighing over a thousand kilos which blocked the last manoeuvre to free the new-born. No bulldozer was available in those dramatic moments and the sad epilogue of the story was emerging with the succession of the atrocious death of an innocent, guilty only of having been born in a country with "controlled seismic risk". The woman petrified by pain seemed to have aged a hundred years in an instant and in the throes of a sort of mediumistic trance, after hearing the umpteenth and last call of her dying puppy, she grabbed that monolithic trunk like a twig and freed the little one who re-emerged from that sea of stones and dust, white with chalk, but alive. Weeping her heroic mother pressed to her chest bringing it back to life once more. This pathetic tale is a clear example of how one can change one's behavioural module in an instant. Often the pragmatic mind is a bad advisor and only a powerful and saving imaginative can save our lives, in the most critical moments. Where the psyche had already provided its negative response, aggravated by the observation of the impossibility of rescue by the military, the heart and maternal instinct had acted as leverage, changing the fate of two human beings in the space of a few seconds, forgetting the Test of the social that gave up the child for doomed, because a trunk of a ton is not a weight that can be lifted under ordinary conditions by anyone... let alone a weak and defenceless woman! The evaluative error in this story was to consider the situation of a mother who is watching her baby die, a normal event. Situations of this kind widely cross the margins of the ordinary and the normal, think that with regard to the dramatic intensity of such suffering, even the Bible states that: “no parent should ever survive the death of a child”, this is because an event of the gender is the source of immense pain that no mother should ever have to suffer. Once the extreme threshold of suffering has been reached, the lever of change is automatically triggered, allowing an extraordinary change in the human physiology of a mother who, lashed by the imminent loss of her child, makes a change that would otherwise not be remotely conceivable or feasible to completely interrupt the vicious circuit. After all, isn’t it true that pain and pleasure shape all our behavioural patterns like ductile clay and through this conditioning allow us to quickly process radical, sensitive and lasting changes. When you have reached the limit, you too can say enough and change your life, in an instant with a simple snap of your fingers, just decide it… If you want to lose weight, stop smoking or drinking alcohol, you too are in a critical situation and you have I've just slipped my head into the noose, but the rope around my neck isn't tightened yet… It's never too late to turn the tables and start another round of a new game, all to be played: the game of your life! Don't wait for certain things to happen before deciding to change walls. Often it is the lack of conviction and certainty that prevents the changes that are actually definitely within your reach, the fear of losing is much stronger than the desire to win. Forget limited and suffocating coordinates to rediscover your time that has been stolen from you, look out of time as in a new Samhain party! You are ready? Arm yourself with patience, courage and trust. Treat yourself to an escape out of time through an internalisation of the eternal tyrant Time! Yes, you read right: Time! Giving time means giving love, since the time generally available is so little for anyone and therefore should be used sparingly. Loving a person means dedicating attention and time to spend in their company. Are not the mythical fairy tales of Sleeping Beauty, Snow White, the love dream of Romeo and Juliet woven into a plot where time escapes like water from a sink without a stopper? You will therefore understand why in a context like this time metaphorically rises to the euphemistic and classic meaning of money and it will therefore be desirable that we learn to value its message as soon as possible, given that often one life is not enough... Another way of growth of the individual is based on the Fire element and makes use of often violent methods to pursue a state of expanded consciousness or super consciousness. This path includes the initiatory techniques based on the violent, sudden and sometimes violent subversion of the ordinary form of thought, as found for example in the school of Rinzai Zen, or of Sudden Enlightenment and therefore on the use of narcotic substances, the famous Herbs of the Power of Castaneda's Don Juan, on Soma, on the practice of tantric sex, Kundalini Yoga, black magical practices in general, some hypnotic practices, etc. These techniques are not free from risks and can induce the adept to lose the right path, blazing in the fire of a change that is too sudden, unexpected and astonishing, raising him above the common human dimension, just as happened in the case of the mother who saves the child from the rubble.

The Ugly Duckling Syndrome

All things are possible to him who believes

Mark 9:23

Nothing in life has absolute value; everything depends on the meaning we choose to give it. That's why we can't ignore the importance of consciously defining our true goals—only then can we truly pursue happiness.

A ski champion, fully equipped with an anorak, boots, and a helmet, can easily conquer a downhill course. But if they decided to run the New York Marathon in the same gear, they'd be at a serious disadvantage. Beyond the amusement their unusual outfit would provoke, their defeat would be inevitable—skiing and running are fundamentally different and incompatible.

Similarly, people often resign themselves to an unfulfilling life simply because they've grown accustomed to it. This doesn't mean you have to be chronically dissatisfied, but rather that you should take an honest moment of self-reflection.

Don't be afraid to ask yourself life's essential questions:

1. Why am I here?
2. What is the purpose of my existence?
3. Am I engaged in something that truly makes me happy?
4. And when I finally achieve what I seek, will it really bring me happiness?

These questions don't require perfect answers, only genuine, instinctive reflection—free from pride and prejudice. Lying to yourself means losing twice!

Just because you've been a banker or an office worker for twenty years doesn't mean you have to be one for the rest of your life, especially if it doesn't make you happy. Stop evaluating the future purely in material terms—listen to the call of your heart, which only longs for joy and freedom.

Don't fear losing a paycheck if it means changing paths. If you're an artist but can't express your creativity in your current job, dare to follow your deepest desires. Life is like a ten-speed bicycle: most people never use all the gears and struggle uphill, while a wide, inviting downhill of bliss awaits them just beyond their hesitation.

Eliminate "if only" from your vocabulary and remove negativity from your most common phrases. Words can be weapons or seeds of joy—choose yours wisely.

And remember: if you don't make time to care for your soul's well-being, you will find time to be sick.

The Story Of Rapunzel

Love the sinner and You hate sin.

Jesus

Like many fairy tales about gnomes and fairies, the story of Rapunzel is a metaphor with a hidden meaning—one that speaks to self-image.

Rapunzel is a young woman imprisoned in a tower by an old witch who constantly tells her how ugly she is. Surrounded by nothing but negativity, she begins to believe it. Her self-image is shaped entirely by the cruel judgments of the envious witch, leaving her sad and hopeless. In such conditions, it becomes incredibly difficult to envision success.

Growing up surrounded by wealth and achievement makes it easy to adopt those patterns. But for those raised in hardship and despair, positive models are scarce, making success seem almost unattainable.

One day, a handsome prince happens to pass by the tower. Seeing Rapunzel at the window, he is captivated by her beauty. Overcome with admiration, he expresses his fascination. For the first time, Rapunzel sees herself reflected in someone else's eyes—

not as the hideous creature the witch described, but as a woman of undeniable beauty. In that moment of newfound awareness, she takes control of her own destiny, lowering her famous golden braid to let him climb up and rescue her.

It was never the tower or the witch that truly imprisoned Rapunzel—it was her own mistaken belief in her unworthiness. Only when she recognized her hidden beauty did she free herself, opening the door to infinite possibilities.

We all, dear readers, must identify the inner witch or wizard that keeps us captive. To do so, examine yourself and see if you recognize any of these self-image issues:

- JEALOUSY
- NEGATIVE OPINIONS ABOUT YOURSELF
- FEELINGS OF GUILT
- INABILITY TO COMPLIMENT OTHERS
- DIFFICULTY ACCEPTING COMPLIMENTS
- NOT VALUING YOUR OWN NEEDS
- FEAR OF ASKING FOR WHAT YOU WANT
- DENYING YOURSELF EVEN SMALL PLEASURES
- STRUGGLING TO EXPRESS AFFECTION
- INABILITY TO RECEIVE AND ENJOY AFFECTION FROM OTHERS

- BEING OVERLY CRITICAL OF OTHERS
- CONSTANTLY COMPARING YOURSELF TO OTHERS
- LIVING IN A STATE OF POOR HEALTH

If you identify with at least three of these, you may be a Rapunzel in need of a self-image transformation. Here, dear "gourmets of the soul," is a simple yet effective therapeutic menu to help you break free from the Ugly Duckling Syndrome:

- ACCEPT COMPLIMENTS: Say thank you, whether the compliment is spontaneous or not—it still holds value.
- GIVE COMPLIMENTS: One of the best ways to feel good about yourself is to recognize beauty in others.
- REWARD YOURSELF: When you achieve something, acknowledge your success and give yourself credit.
- SEPARATE YOUR BELIEFS FROM YOUR WORTH: Your mistakes don't define you. If you accidentally bump into someone's car at a red light, it doesn't mean you're a terrible person—it just means you made a mistake. Forgive yourself!
- TREAT YOUR BODY WELL: It's the only one you have (unless cloning takes off), and everything you eat, drink, think, or breathe affects it. Care for it wisely!
- SHOW OTHERS HOW YOU WANT TO BE TREATED: Lead by example in how you treat them, and set clear boundaries.

- SURROUND YOURSELF WITH GOOD PEOPLE.
- WORK WITH JOY, WITHOUT GUILT: Use positive affirmations.
- CONSUME POSITIVE CONTENT: Read books, watch movies, and listen to music that inspire you.
- VISUALIZE YOUR BEST SELF: Picture yourself as healthier, happier, more confident whatever you aspire to be. Your thoughts shape your reality, so make them beautiful.

Change isn't easy—if it were, everyone would be content and happy. But in the duality of life, struggle makes joy meaningful. A negative self-image is self-perpetuating, and the moment you start to change, you may find yourself slipping into old patterns of self-blame and doubt.

But keep going. When you start following this soul-nourishing "diet" and the guidance we offer as your coaches, you'll see results. Sparks will fly—of joy, of course!

Depression:
Disease Of The Soul

Nothing grand was ever achieved
without the enthusiasm!

Ralph.R.W. Emerson

The COVID-19 epidemic has triggered a 25% increase in the prevalence of anxiety and depression worldwide, and even after more than five years since its outbreak, its impact continues to reverberate. Among COVID-19 survivors, psychopathological implications such as depression, anxiety, and cognitive impairments are now recognized as key symptoms of "post-acute COVID-19 syndrome." Studies indicate that approximately 35% of patients experience depressive symptoms at short-, medium-, and long-term follow-ups after contracting the Severe Acute Respiratory Syndrome Coronavirus-2 (SARS-CoV-2) infection.

Post-COVID-19 depression exacerbates fatigue and impairs neurocognitive functioning, sleep quality, overall well-being, and daily life activities. The underlying mechanisms behind these symptoms are primarily linked to inflammation triggered by the immune response to the virus, as well as the persistent psychological burden experienced during and after infection. Given the vast number of SARS-CoV-2-infected individuals and the high incidence of post-COVID-19 depression, there is a growing concern that depressive disorders will become even more widespread. Addressing this issue requires proactive screening, accurate diagnosis, targeted treatment, and continuous monitoring of mental health among COVID-19 survivors to mitigate the burden of depression and the years of life lost to disability. This paper reviews the current literature to synthesize available evidence on the epidemiology, clinical manifestations, neurobiological mechanisms, and pharmacological treatment of post-COVID-19 depressive symptoms. (Source: PubMed, Mario Gennaro Mazza et al., CNS Drugs, July 2022.)

The impulse to embark on an alchemical and introspective journey toward self-discovery often arises from a subtle yet persistent sense of dissatisfaction—one that can render even the most mundane aspects of life uncomfortable or unfulfilling. This nebulous feeling of existential futility lingers, leaving important life questions unanswered.

To the untrained eye, these early signs might be mistaken for a generic, almost trivial, form of depression. However, they are anything but ordinary and certainly do not deserve to be numbed by a cocktail of benzodiazepines. Rather, they should be acknowledged, examined, and interpreted with care.

Fortunately, nature is generous. If you pay close attention, you will find the remedy to your suffering hidden in plain sight. It may be embedded in the words of a friend, disguised within the lines of a book you once dismissed as dull, or even lurking in an unexpected piece of wisdom from a relative whose presence you barely tolerated at a holiday gathering.

In short, when life leaves you stranded with a flat tire, don't despair—search a little deeper, and you'll find your spare. Just be mindful: you may know where your journey begins, but its destination remains uncertain. So abandon rigid plans and set forth with the simple joy of exploration in your heart. Because, ultimately, the real reward is the journey itself—the act of being, of running simply for the pleasure of running, much like the eagle soars solely for the joy of flight. Shedding the weight of the ego makes the journey lighter and more fluid.

I have witnessed individuals so entangled in their own egos—grander than cathedrals—that they perished rather than change their lifestyle habits. Conversely, I have seen humble souls rise like a phoenix from the ashes of dire conditions: cancer, rheumatoid arthritis, multiple sclerosis, and beyond.

The illusion of the ego often leads people to seek solace in fleeting indulgences—money, unbridled pleasure, luxury cars, extravagant attire, lavish feasts—all while obscuring the true self, the diamond buried deep within. Misused wealth suffocates the essential, yet paradoxically, poverty does not always foster spirituality. As Deepak Chopra suggests, the poor are often forced to think about money even more than the wealthy, simply for survival.

Only a society freed from economic distress and time scarcity can truly aspire to the ideal of well-being—a modern vision of the Welfare State that aligns with the pursuit of quality of life, a goal championed by contemporary humanitarian movements rising from the remnants of historical materialism.

When humanity finally unlocks its inner potential, awakening the true self, it will gain the ability to fully interpret both life and soul, embracing its divine cosmic blueprint and achieving harmony between body and mind. When well-being becomes accessible to all, when people can reclaim their existential dignity through conscious choices, then—perhaps—the Celestial Jerusalem, long sought by poets and visionaries, will reappear in all its brilliance within every heart.

The age of conflict and suffering, foretold in the sacred Vedic texts as "Kali Yuga," is poised to give way to a new paradigm of unity, expanded consciousness, and personal transformation. This era is upon us, and whether we accept it or not, we are all its protagonists.

How much time have we wasted searching outside ourselves for what has always been within?

Is this not the essence of the Labors of Hercules—the timeless myth that echoes through the twilight of human consciousness? That relentless, hidden will to live, propelling us forward despite the fragility of existence, urging us to persist at all costs.

There is no beginning of anything
Nor any stopping the motion of anything
Realizing this is the perfection of wisdom.
(Prajinaparti)

Homo Hominis Medicus: Dream Elixir Of The Soul

It is not impossible, metaphysically speaking, that there is
a continuous and lasting dream like the life of a man...
But assuming that the phenomena are related, it doesn't matter
whether they are called dreams or not,
for experience shows that one is not deceived
to the extent that phenomena are learned,
when they are apprehended according to the truths of reason
Leibniz (Nouw.Ess.IV, 2,14)

Philosophers have long used dreams to illustrate the uncertainty of distinguishing between dreaming and waking life, employing them as an instrument of theoretical doubt.

Yet, if the human organism—just as it produces bile or hemoglobin—can generate the dreams of the night, why should it not also create the ideas of the day? Life and dreams are but frames of the same film, to paraphrase Schopenhauer.

Are you truly awake? And if not, how can you awaken the traveler within? How can you rediscover the Eden from which you were expelled?

The first demand man must make of himself is to become the leading actor, director, and producer of his own alchemical rebirth—an effective synonym for healing through inner awakening. After all, man is the only true medicine for himself.

To accept the necessity of awakening is to accept the existence of dreams, much like the paradox of the liar by Eubulides of Miletus. Suppose I say: "I am lying." Since lying means stating a falsehood, my claim is true only if it is false.

An intriguing anecdote about the tailcoat suggests that a waiter is a man who wears a tailcoat without anyone noticing it. Conversely, some men appear to be waiters the moment they don a tailcoat. In both cases, the tailcoat itself holds no inherent value.

The paradox of dream and life thus forms an intriguing equation, one that the challenge of human incarnation presents to your vigilant souls.

"Homo hominis medicus," argued the Latin fathers, and we stand with them: only man can come to the aid of another man by rediscovering his own Parakletos—his inner healer—who, though perhaps dormant, slumbers within each of us.

Listening to the genie of the lamp, one learns that the true source of anguish and illness lies in the rigidity of behavioral patterns to which one is subjugated, blocking individual evolutionary perspectives.

When a human being abandons his visions and ceases to build castles in the air—suffocating the child within—he severs the lifeblood that enlivens him, transforming into what Americans, with a grim sense of noir, describe as a "dead man walking."

William Shakespeare, who understood many of the secrets of the human soul, writes in *The Tempest* (Act IV, Scene I): "We are such stuff as dreams are made on." Yet, man seems to have lost the habit of dreaming and, in doing so, has misplaced the key to the Garden of Eden, where life was a dream, and the dream was life.

The rampant use of drugs such as benzodiazepines and antidepressants to quell the torments of the soul is burying the true self beneath the oppressive ego of an encroaching pharmacocracy. The collective unconscious has been robbed of its dreams, left adrift in the dark waves of a civilization at the turn of the millennium. Will the man of the third millennium be able to reclaim them?

Dreams are the true elixir of the soul, allowing it to glide on a soft carpet across parallel universes and infinite dimensions, where the coordinates of space and time dissolve like snow in the spring rain.

Emotions are cumulative, and when they reach a critical mass, they explode like a bolt from the blue, producing overwhelming and unexpected results. Often, a single fateful moment—an insignificant mishap—can trigger this massive eruption.

Only in dreams is man granted shelter from the tempests of existence. Only in this ethereal state is he permitted, if only for a fleeting moment, to taste his divine nature. And only through the dissolution of the mind in this pantomime of reincarnations can he return to the Inner Absolute, which, in the etymology of traditional India, is condensed into a single, unifying word: *Atman*.

Freezing one's perspectives means blocking one's divine inner creative power. Every time a human being experiences an emotional conflict, it is added to the catalogue of previous wounds, stored in the vast archive of subjective suffering. The mind meticulously records, categorizes, and cross-references these experiences, filing them away in the subconscious, ready to resurface when triggered by similar circumstances.

This ever-growing volume of unresolved emotions forms a true Neuro-Emotional Complex, much like a cork in a bottle of Cabernet. Every time you attempt to pour more wine, the cork resurfaces, threatening to taint your nectar. Likewise, past wounds, seemingly rationally resolved but still subconsciously reactive, re-emerge in times of stress, obstructing true healing and transformation.

A similar mechanism was observed in Plato's *Tabula Rasa*, an expression sometimes used to describe the soul's state before acquiring knowledge. The ability to store and process such experiences is conditioned by numerous factors—nutritional, genetic, emotional, and environmental—that interact in unique ways within each individual.

When the burden of these accumulated memories becomes too heavy, protective disengagement mechanisms automatically trigger neurovegetative alarms, manifesting as premonitory symptoms governed by the Sympathetic Autonomic Nervous System. If left unaddressed, these signals can evolve into overt disease.

The activation of the sympathetic nervous system is a crucial survival mechanism in emergencies, but it becomes costly and detrimental when perpetuated in non-life-threatening situations. It is akin to taking out a high-interest loan—it may provide temporary relief, but over time, the accumulated interest can far exceed the principal amount, leading to disastrous consequences.

Preventing this state of red alert is the cornerstone of any true orthomolecular healing.

To know oneself and to respect oneself is the first requirement for respecting others and cultivating responsible individuals who can be entrusted with the future of the planet. Loving oneself is, in truth, a simple act—one that requires dedicating time to oneself and to others.

After all, to love is to give time to someone. And that is precisely what we are doing right now.

Panfhealing® hopes to help you recognize and prevent such risk situations—or, when unavoidable, to navigate them with due caution—returning to you the time you had lost.

The proposed treatments aim precisely at preventing the old hard drive of memory from rebooting with each new emotional conflict, preventing it from jamming on the grooves of past wounds and recreating stagnant, repetitive cycles that hinder true liberation from stress and suffering.

New Atlantis: Requiem For A Vanished Civilization

The Big Bang occurred 16 billion years ago, more precisely on April 12 at 3pm.
It was raining, but the planets had still decided to go for a walk.
Since that primordial explosion, the universe has continued to expand continuously at sidereal speed and even today they are trying to figure out who left the gas on.

(Francesco Salvi, History of World Culture, Mondadori publisher)

There exists a religion older than Christianity, one that has transmitted essential values for the evolution of humanity—love, justice, forgiveness, and the search for truth. This is the wisdom of the Vedas (*vid*, from the ancient Sanskrit, meaning "knowledge of the Supreme"). From the vast ocean of Vedic wisdom, the great religions have descended and to it, they inevitably return.

Historically, the Vedas represent the oldest known books of knowledge on the planet. They are not easy texts to interpret, nor are they confined to any single, well-defined space. Their influence permeates the entire cosmos, existing as an immense and sacred repository of wisdom, transcribed at least 6,000 years ago—though undoubtedly far older—by the sage Vyasa. It was he who compiled and commented on these texts in his monumental work, the *Srimad Bhagavatam*.

This knowledge was likely transmitted for millennia through an esoteric and oral tradition, employing mythological symbolism and allegory to preserve its original purity and shield it from the inevitable distortions of political and social interference.

Exegetical sources suggest that the origins of the Vedas may trace back to the migrations of the Aryan peoples, who journeyed from the European coasts to the Tibetan plateau and the Himalayan mountain ranges some 900,000 years ago. Even biblical sources speak of the Arys reaching the Caucasus before splitting into three great migratory waves, spreading civilization from the banks of the Nile to the Indus Valley.

Originally, all planetary knowledge was said to be contained within a single, unified Vedic tome—a monumental work exploring the divine presence hidden behind the veil of the phenomenal world, spanning theology, philosophy, metaphysics, and more. One can only imagine its colossal scope—far surpassing the *Encyclopaedia*

Britannica, the Library of Congress, or even the endless sprawl of Wikipedia has ever generated.

It was then that Vyasa, with great foresight (and perhaps some editorial wisdom), took pity on future scholars. Like a visionary publisher releasing a serial publication, he decided to break the work into installments—an ancient equivalent of the *Merck Manual* or the *MSD Medical Encyclopedia of Health*—thus making its wisdom more accessible.

He divided the knowledge into four fundamental texts:

- **RIG VEDA**: The cornerstone of Vedic mythology, comprising ten extensive volumes known as the *Mandalas*.
- **YAJUR VEDA**: A compendium of sacrificial formulas used by priests in ritual ceremonies.
- **SAMA VEDA**: A collection of mantras, chants, and melodies, deeply cryptic and imbued with initiatory meaning.
- **ATHARVA VEDA**: A work concerning psychic powers and extrasensory perception—let's hope our politicians never get their hands on it, or we'd have more than enough trouble. This text, compiled in twenty volumes, contains mystical words of power and esoteric knowledge capable of transcending the known four-dimensional reality.

To complement these foundational texts, the *Upanishads* serve as philosophical reflections and epilogues to the Vedic teachings. Originally, there were said to be 1,180 Upanishads. Today, according to Sai Baba, only 108 remain. But who knows? In some secluded monastery in Tibet or elsewhere, fragments of the lost volumes may still be safeguarded, handed down ritually through prayer and meditation.

Plato, an intellectual of rare caliber, immersed himself in the company of great sages such as Socrates. It is likely that he had access—if only in glimpses—to the sacred Vedic texts, drawing from them the philosophical insights that echo through his *Timaeus*.

In this work, he recounts the story of an Egyptian priest of the goddess Sais, who revealed to Solon the ancient tale of Atlantis—an island beyond the fabled Pillars of Hercules, lost to the memory of mankind after the Great Flood.

Atlantis, in this account, was a wise and enlightened monarchy that reigned unchallenged from Libya to Egypt and from Europe to Etruria. Its people lived in harmony, much like the utopias found in the most beautiful fairy tales.

The civilization of Atlantis was highly advanced, particularly in its mastery of crystal and stone technologies for energy and healing purposes. Some researchers speculate that Nikola Tesla's revolutionary discoveries were inspired by this lost knowledge. Yet, as with all technological marvels, these powers could be wielded for good or for destruction. Tragically, the Atlanteans succumbed to their own hubris, signing the death warrant of their golden age.

Like all great civilizations, Atlantis bore within it the seed of its own downfall. The insatiable lust for power and the unchecked ambitions of its ruling priestly caste led to a cosmic delusion of omnipotence. Dissatisfied with their vast dominion, they began to abuse their technologies, forgetting their sacred duty to respect Mother Earth. Reckless experiments in warfare and energy manipulation ensued, destabilizing the natural balance.

During this period, it is said that much of the energy harnessed through their crystals dissipated into the earth, while discord and rivalry infiltrated the ranks of their leaders. Their imperial ambitions led them to attempt the conquest of Athens—a seemingly unassuming city-state that, against all odds, fiercely resisted and ultimately secured its freedom from this towering war machine.

It was then that Atlantis, once invincible, began to show signs of decay. A profound, irreversible political, structural, and geobiological crisis took hold. Perhaps some among the priestly class foresaw the impending catastrophe. Recognizing the imminent collapse, a few enlightened souls sought to safeguard their vast knowledge, ensuring it would not be lost to oblivion. They carried their sacred wisdom to the corners of the world, planting the seeds of civilization in lands that would one day flourish—among them, Egypt and Tibet.

But the island itself, doomed by the abuse of its own power and the folly of its rulers, succumbed to the waves. In an instant, it was swallowed by the ocean, leaving behind only legends and an uncharted abyss where once it had stood.

And now, as history marches forward, one cannot help but wonder: Will the civilization of the island of Europe meet a similar fate? Will it one day be reduced to a mere footnote—a brief *Elzevir*, scarcely longer than a few columns in a provincial newspaper, relegated to the fading margins of time?

New Age And Next Age

"O my master! O my master!
O you who destroy
But without being cruel!
You who build
without however being good!
You who were before time,
and you are not old!
You who cover everything like the sky,
that like earth you support everything,
that you are the author of everything
without being skilled (spontaneous activity)!
Understanding you thus is heavenly bliss."

"O my master! O my master!
You who destroy—yet not with cruelty.
You who build—yet not out of kindness.
You who existed before time—yet are not old.
You who cover all like the sky,
And support all like the earth.
You, the source of all things—

Yet untrained, spontaneous!
To understand you thus is heavenly bliss."

See which one it's better

Chuang Tzu

Lieh-Tzu, one of the founding fathers of Taoism (along with Chuang-Tzu and Lao-Tzu, *E/n*), argued that it is futile to speak of the Principle to the arrogant and the violent. Such individuals lack the necessary qualities to comprehend it; their flaws prevent them from receiving wisdom and benefiting from guidance. These paradoxes reflect the Taoist belief in the natural, effortless flow of the universe, where actions occur spontaneously and harmoniously without intentional force or intervention.

The fundamental prerequisite for teaching is that the student must acknowledge that they do *not* already know everything—after all, one cannot fill a bottle that is already full.

Age is never an obstacle to learning, just as raw intelligence alone is not always the most effective tool in the pursuit of knowledge. What truly matters, beyond the teacher's willingness to transmit wisdom with love and for the growth of both the individual and the community, is the student's curiosity and humble openness to continuous learning.

There is an old tale about an artist from the Song dynasty who spent three years carving a life-sized mulberry leaf in jade for his prince. Upon seeing it, Lieh-Tzu remarked: *"If nature took as long, trees would have very few leaves."*

So too, in the transmission of doctrine, the sage relies on the intrinsic power of truth, not on artificial craftsmanship.

In reality, the true past—the one told in non-linear ways—exerts such an overwhelming influence on the mind that it can stifle fresh and creative responses. As the Italian philosopher and historian Giambattista Vico observed, history moves in cycles of peaks and valleys, with everything repeating itself in different forms. Nothing genuinely new appears on the observer's horizon, only variations of patterns already set in motion.

The sudden and violent downfall of political regimes, or the radical transformation of cultural paradigms, is often catalyzed by changes in the medium of information. Never before has this been as true as it is today.

Like revolution, *fashion* serves as a vehicle for introducing new attitudes, beliefs, and behaviours into the institutional frameworks of a society—whether within an individual, a nation, or an entire civilization. Through rapid communication and widespread assimilation, social trends accelerate the acceptance of ideas that, without this mechanism, would take far longer to gain traction.

To dismiss this so-called "New Era" as nothing more than a passing trend would be simplistic and misguided. History reminds us that *Cartesianism, the Enlightenment, Newtonian physics, Darwinism, Positivism (as formulated by Auguste Comte), Idealism, Neo-Idealism, and Pragmatism*—all of these were, in their time, intellectual *fashions*. And yet, each of them played a decisive role in shaping the history of culture.

The movement known as *New Age* emerged synergistically in 1962 in Findhorn, Scotland, and took root in California during the 1960s and '70s. In a society increasingly shaped by materialistic values, many young people found themselves longing for something more—something deeper. This yearning for freedom and transformation found its most radical expression in the *Hippie* movement, a rejection of rigid social and political control structures.

At the time, cultural outlets were scarce, and the counterculture movement filled an intellectual and spiritual void that modern media had yet to address. Today, such a revolution would take an entirely different form—it would not rely on communal gatherings in parks or mass protests on the streets but would unfold across websites, social media platforms, and digital activism. Instead of unfurling a banner beneath the United Nations building, protestors would likely draft a viral message directed at world peace delegates.

Yet, beneath its anti-establishment veneer, the *New Age* was driven by a profound mystical quest—an exploration of altered states of consciousness and reality, a celebration of individual creativity. However, this pursuit was often conflated with the chemically induced expansion of perception, achieved not through meditative discipline but through hallucinogenic substances, inhaled or injected.

Even leading scholars of psychology, such as Timothy Leary of Harvard, advocated for lysergic acid (LSD) as a tool for breaking mental barriers. Meanwhile, peyote and mescaline were celebrated as vehicles for perceiving and expressing *psychedelic art*.

Music, too, became a powerful medium for amplifying the ideals and aspirations of the era. Among the most influential prophets of this cultural shift were the *Beatles*—the legendary quartet from Liverpool—who bridged the gap between East and West. Their exploration of Indian spirituality and philosophy laid the groundwork for the modern diffusion of universalist ideas, including those found in the *Theosophy* of Helena Petrovna Blavatsky.

And so, here we are.

Welcome to the future—because you are already there.

The Pillars Of Hercules

"Tell him for me to reverse direction
and then retrace the entire circle,
then he will find what he seeks.
Watch his steps,
and when he has an open heart,
sharp mind and skillful hands.... then bring it to me"

Alice A. Bailey – The Labors of Hercules

This book could not be considered complete without at least a brief exploration of the vital role of the spine. As both an orthopedic surgeon and a kinesiologist, I have long regarded this anatomical structure as fundamental, and I feel compelled to share some reflections on the subject.

By analogy with the legendary *Pillars of Hercules*—the boundary beyond which ancient civilizations' expansionist ambitions faltered—the spine too represents a relatively unexplored and cryptic frontier.

Great credit is due to G. Goodhart, the pioneer of modern kinesiology, who rightly emphasized the spine's significance as a *reservoir* for the accumulation and distribution of information flowing to and from the external world. His groundbreaking work placed particular focus on *vertebral subluxation*—a misalignment that, despite not reaching the threshold of full dislocation, can profoundly disrupt the body's energy flow and overall function.

The spine is far more than a static scaffold upon which muscles, tendons, and nerves are suspended. It is a dynamic, intelligent structure—a *microcosm* within the *macrocosm* of an individual's life.

Postural habits, positions, and movement patterns are deeply intertwined with the psychological and emotional tensions a person experiences. When someone suffers from *lumbago*, *stiff neck*, or *cervical pain*, these are not mere mechanical inconveniences but rather somatic expressions of deeper existential conflicts. The spine functions as a *black box*—absorbing, storing, and encoding life's stressors with more precision than the most sophisticated of computers. Rigidity, excessive muscular tension, or loss of flexibility are not random occurrences; they are physical manifestations of stagnation, a reflection of an individual's struggle to navigate and resolve inner conflicts.

A growing number of orthopedic specialists are beginning to recognize kinesiology as a bloodless, non-invasive solution to conditions that, in the past, would have been addressed almost exclusively through spinal surgery.

Beyond its biomechanical functions, the spine serves as a faithful indicator of a person's natural talents, emotional state, and level of self-awareness. It operates as a *body-mind syncytium*, shaping the way an individual processes experiences and responds to external stimuli. Just as the mast of a sailboat provides stability in both turbulent and tranquil waters, so too does the spine enable a person to navigate the vast ocean of awareness.

The loss of even a single vertebral joint's full range of motion does not merely restrict mechanical function—it can compromise the body's overall vitality, subtly yet powerfully disrupting the flow of *subtle energies*. This, in turn, conditions mental, emotional, and even spiritual capacity, limiting an individual's ability to attune to certain frequencies of their total reality.

A blocked vertebra can mean far more than a localized stiffness—it can signify a deep internal stagnation, predisposing the individual to suffering and disease.

Vertebrae-Organs-Meridian Correlations And Emotions

Organ / Meridian	Vertebrae Involved	Correlated Emotions
Stomach	T8, T10, T12	Excessive stress, acidosis
Spleen	T1, T5, T9	Poor self-esteem
Pancreas	L5	—
Large Intestine	L5	Dogmatic positions
Lung	T1, T8, L2 (left) T2, T9, L3 (right)	Feeling doomed
Bladder	L5	Willpower paralyzed
Kidney	T1, T5, T8	Fear
Gallbladder	T4	Resentment
Liver	T2, T5, T8	Anger
Intestine	L5	Vulnerability, abandonment
Heart	T2, T8, T12	Excessive emotions
Thyroid	C1, C4, C7	Emotional instability, paranoia
Adrenals	T7, T9, T11	—
Prostate	L5	—

Testicles	Sacroiliac joints	—
Ovaries	L3, L5	Aboulia, total exhaustion
Uterus	Coccyx	—
Pituitary	C2, C5, T1	—

The recurring nature of symptoms and pain in the same anatomical areas—be it the familiar back pain, the usual neck stiffness, chronic colitis, persistent bronchitis, or seasonal allergies—suggests that mind, body, and soul are often segregated in their perspectives. Episodic or recurrent disorders, like those outlined in the diagram, are frequently linked to vertebral misalignments and subluxations.

It's common to witness a tendency to dwell in self-pity, where symptoms and illnesses are almost celebrated, as though they were the culprits of dissatisfaction and unmet desires, instead of being the effects of deeper, unresolved failures and frustrations.

Miraculous healings often occur when subluxated vertebrae are realigned and regain their harmonious position, thus freeing the nervous system from the restrictive patterns that had previously held it captive. This process, during Panfhealing ®, can sometimes be accompanied by a liberating release of tears, which not only signifies the mind-body-soul syncytium's rapid reorganization but also correlates with a decrease in tissue acidity. The stress associated with vertebral subluxations is alleviated, and once realigned, the body can quickly begin to re-alkalize its tissues.

Healing is intrinsically tied to the physiological alkalization of the body. The presence of excessive organic acid radicals often creates an insurmountable barrier to restoring the balance needed for complete recovery. In such cases, it is vital to inform the patient about improving their dietary and water intake habits.

A helpful guideline is to ensure that at least 50% of one's daily food intake consists of vegetables (with at least one-third being raw), 20% from fruit, and the remaining 30% should be split equally between cereals, seeds, sprouts, healthy fats, and animal proteins—though animal proteins should not exceed 5-7% of the total daily intake.

Additionally, it is crucial to drink at least 2 liters of water a day, with a fixed mineral residue of less than 50 mg/l and a pH between 5.9 and 6.5. This amount should be increased for individuals who engage in sports or activities involving intense sweating.

Patients often report that the feeling after neuro-emotional unblocking is akin to wiping the dust and mud from a windshield while driving or listening to a beautiful classical piece, such as Pachelbel's Canon or David Bailey's piano arrangements. The use of alkalizing music during Panfhealing® can significantly facilitate the process of releasing repressed emotions.

The Bridge Emotions (E.P.):

You can manipulate your emotions and moods
in an instant, just like you change your clothes,
just as in your worst enemy you can discover your best master!
Thank him what are you waiting for?

– Free communication

Like an old wounded elephant that never forgets, the human subconscious clings to every slight, every wound—physical, emotional, verbal—from both pre- and postnatal life. Emotional conflicts in humans are cumulative. Just like compound interest in a bank account, they grow over time. The psychological investment of energy—our emotional drive toward people, goals, fantasies, ideas, or even toward ourselves—is known as *cathexis* (from the Greek *katecho*, meaning "to hold" or "to occupy").

Every new conflict we experience is automatically cross-referenced with past emotional imprints, layering and compounding them like a snowflake gathering mass as it slides down the slope of life—eventually becoming an emotional avalanche that can sweep away everything in its path.

When someone experiences an insult, an act of violence, or verbal aggression, it leaves a deep imprint in the subconscious. These negative emotional residues can resurface when least expected, triggering physiological defense responses—almost like an internal alarm system sounding off in the body's sensory matrix.

The subconscious doesn't rationalize; it reacts. It stores these painful experiences through cathexis—as emotional "packages" of energy tied to specific memories and physiological states. When a similar memory or idea is recalled, the emotional and metabolic context from the original event is instantly reactivated.

The Central Nervous System (CNS), through the Reticular Activating System (RAS), functions like an emotional filter. It captures emotionally charged input from the environment and from memory—then amplifies and replays this input in critical moments, showing up as anxiety, irritation, sadness, resentment—or, conversely, as motivation, gratitude, joy, and inner strength.

In any given moment, we're bombarded with a staggering number of sensory inputs. Yet the brain can only process a tiny sliver of that data. Through its filtering network (the reason it's called "reticular"), only the information deemed personally relevant slips through—like selected fish caught in the net of subjective reality.

Just think of two football teams playing in a roaring stadium. Each team hears the encouragement of their own fans and largely filters out the noise of their opponents' supporters. That selective listening? Pure RAS in action.

Under the label E.P. (Emotional Programs), we refer to those emotions and feelings that, although deeply personal and subjective, wield immense influence over both mind and body. These emotions build a sort of bridge between the psyche and the soma. But it's not just pain that shapes us—opposing emotions like love, trust, gratitude, and admiration can also form powerful positive anchors, launching us toward fulfillment and joy.

Truly healthy, successful people tend to harness this form of emotional self-programming. They don't shame or ignore their symptoms and emotional reactions—instead, they view them as precious signals, not enemies. Trying to resist emotions is like trying to stop an avalanche with a teaspoon. A far wiser approach is to learn how to listen—genuinely listen—to what the body is trying to say through its emotions.

Emotions are like buoys in a sailing race: they're pivot points that mark where we've been, and help us steer toward where we need to go. For instance, a traumatic betrayal in love might lead someone to seek a future partner with completely opposite traits—gentler, calmer, more nurturing. That's not necessarily a reflection of their authentic desires, but often a defensive counter-reaction. Likewise, those raised in an environment of trust, emotional openness, and healthy communication often unconsciously seek partners who resonate with that same dynamic.

But here's the kicker: this emotional matching process isn't always based on genuine compatibility. Sometimes it's driven by unresolved pain. Choosing a calm, conflict-free partner might not reflect real chemistry, but rather a knee-jerk response to past trauma. And that mismatch can lead to even deeper dissatisfaction.

That's why in Panfhealing® , we work to bring these buried conflicts and emotional residues to the surface. When acknowledged and processed, they can dissolve—like snow melting in the sun. By cultivating deeper self-awareness, we help people reconstruct the foundations of their emotional strategies, and create lives that reflect who they truly are—not just who they had to be to survive.

Because repressed emotions don't just affect your mood—they can undermine your entire health. The impressions left on your subconscious have the power to shape your world. And yes, that includes your well-being.

The Emotions That Make You Sick Are The Same That Can Save You (Practical Exercise)

Man needs rice as an outlet valve,
animals are not, because they are generally subjected to less mental stress,
not being inclined to become embittered or worn out by a given situation;
In fact, they do not feel guilty or overwhelmed by psychological responsibilities.
In short, they live from day to day and...
most importantly, they don't have weird people in government!

– Panfhealing® Internal orthomolecular training course

The feelings, emotions, and words that weigh us down—those dark visitors of the soul—should never be ignored. Instead, we must listen. They come bearing messages, and no matter how uncomfortable or unwelcome they may seem, they deserve to be heard and examined.

Too often, the sheer intensity of emotional pain blinds us to the deeper, almost *esoteric* wisdom hidden within it. And in doing so, we miss yet another sacred opportunity for personal—and perhaps karmic—growth. But what if we saw these emotions not as enemies, but as guides?

Treat these somber sisters like precious compasses on a foggy, moonless night. Let them point you toward the safest path. But beware: underestimate them, and they may quietly erode your future. Instead, sign a truce. Offer them respect, not resistance. Welcome them like wise old teachers, and you may discover that from the bitterest of musts, you can distill the sweetest wine of joy.

How? By finding the silver lining hidden in the darkest of human experiences:

- **HATE**
- **FEAR**
- **CRITICISM**
- **ANGER**
- **RESENTMENT**
- **ENVY**
- **FRUSTRATION**
- **GUILT**
- **IMPOSED SOLITUDE**
- **ANXIETY**

- **DOUBT**
- **JEALOUSY**
- **SELFISHNESS**
- **BULLYING**

Your Turn: A Home Exercise

Grab a pen and a piece of paper.

Yes, right now.

Start by writing—freely, without structure or judgment—a list of the negative emotions that come to mind. Don't overthink. Let them flow straight from your heart, through your pen, onto the page. No editing. No filter. Just raw honesty. Give yourself five minutes.

Ready?

Go.

Time's up. You did it. Now comes the real alchemy.

Next to each emotion you wrote down, write the positive lesson you've extracted from it—even if it came at a high cost. Think of how you grew, what you learned, or how that pain shaped your strength, your empathy, or your boundaries.

Let it hurt a little—that means you're doing it right.

Now, photocopy that page ten times. Scatter those copies throughout your world—tuck one in your bag, another in your journal, one on the fridge, another on your bathroom mirror. Slip one inside your car's windshield—so you can glance at it in the still moments, while the engine warms up or between red lights.

Do this for a month.

Then, repeat the same exercise. You'll likely discover that the emotional sting has dulled. You'll feel something new—a quiet satisfaction, a sense of mastery. Because you, dear reader, will have reprogrammed your subconscious. You'll have trained your emotional reflexes to be more elastic, more compassionate, and more resilient.

Well done.

We're truly proud of you.

The Chemistry Of Fear

We don't fear all evils,

but only those who can adduce

great pains and destructions

and even these only if they are not too far away

but appear near and imminent.

Aristotle (Rhetoric, II, 5, 1382a 20 ff)

Too bad Aristotle isn't around anymore—he'd have made a top-tier inductee into the Orthomolecular Medicine Hall of Fame. His take on fear remains, in our view, one of the most profound ever expressed in the realms of philosophy and medicine. People don't generally fear things that are far off—everyone knows they'll die eventually. But until death feels close, they don't really give it much thought.

Fear, however, is the real shadow cast over humanity's suffering.

It teams up with anxiety and even excitement to become one of those forces capable of abruptly hijacking human behavior—often for the worse. Still, there's a strange antidote to fear, a kind of emotional anesthesia: the conditions that make danger seem distant or even nonexistent. Wealth, strength, power, and a strong social circle often convince people they're untouchable. Suddenly, they're bold, reckless, even dismissive of real threats.

Think about how many wildly successful people came from lives of poverty, hunger, and pain. The sheer *fear* of going back to that suffering becomes the leverage that propels them to the top. Take Mike Tyson, for example. He grew up in brutal conditions—a troubled kid in and out of juvenile homes and, eventually, prison. The constant need to survive forced him to develop new strategies just to avoid more suffering.

What made Tyson a champion wasn't just talent. It was his ability to channel his aggression—born from the terror of living a life like those around him—into a ferocious drive to change his destiny. He didn't want to *cope* with pain; he wanted to *reprogram* the physiology of suffering itself.

But something changed when comfort came knocking. Fame, money, and excess dulled his hunger. The raw edge of fear that once drove him became blunted. He wasn't the same animal who fought his way out of the Bronx.

What sports journalists often oversimplify as "hunger" is actually one of the deepest motivators in the human psyche.

It's a primal trigger that can awaken hidden instincts—the kind that override fear and fuel transformation.

Fear and pain are tightly linked, as Plato pointed out in the *Philebus*. Pain arises when the delicate balance of the body's internal elements is threatened. Pleasure, on the other hand, is what we feel when that balance is restored.

From a medical standpoint, fear is a red alert that activates our most primitive survival system: the sympathetic nervous system. This system floods our bloodstream with war-ready neurotransmitters and acidifying hormones like adrenaline and noradrenaline—biochemical messengers that gear us up for battle.

But after the fight comes the crash. The body needs to recover and restore its equilibrium. That's when the parasympathetic nervous system kicks in, helping us recharge through rest, sleep, and even moments of temporary depression. It's all part of the cycle.

Interestingly, fear can trigger both systems at once—*sympathetic* and *parasympathetic*—as outlined in Guyton's *Textbook of Medical Physiology* (6th ed., p. 218). Too much tissue acidity tips the balance toward a sympathetic "fight or flight" response. Recovery periods, on the other hand, can shift us toward vagotonia, a parasympathetic state associated with repair and rest.

Here's the kicker: the human body is fundamentally designed to function in an alkaline state. Acidosis—the kind that comes from stress, overtraining, or chronic fear—is an emergency mode. The only organ that breaks this alkaline rule? The stomach, which naturally secretes hydrochloric acid and pepsin to handle digestion.

To keep our bodies running smoothly, we need to respect this design. Life, movement, and stress all produce acidifying byproducts—like lactic acid from muscle fatigue. Interestingly, acidic fruits leave behind alkaline ashes after digestion, while meats and proteins, though structurally alkaline, leave behind acidic ashes.

Now, here's a crucial biological limitation: Humans don't produce the enzyme uricase, which means we struggle to break down uric acid. Our kidneys alone can't handle the overload of toxins this produces. That's why keeping your system as alkaline as possible isn't just trendy wellness advice—it's smart biology. It helps preserve kidney function and promotes optimal health.

Nature has a brilliant way of managing pH balance—but it's a delicate act. Even the tiniest variations in acidity can throw off cellular function, especially since enzymes are incredibly sensitive to these shifts.

Bottom line?

Fear may be a survival mechanism, but understanding and mastering the biochemical terrain it creates is one of the most powerful health strategies we've got.

Effects of Autonomic Nervous System Stimulation

Organ/Function	**Sympathetic Stimulation (Adrenergic)**	**Parasympathetic Stimulation (Cholinergic)**
Eye: Pupil	Dilation (mydriasis) – far vision	Constriction (miosis) – near vision
Eye: Ciliary Muscle	Relaxation – facilitates far vision	Contraction – facilitates near vision
Nasal Glands	Vasoconstriction, reduced secretion	Copious fluid secretion
Lacrimal Glands (Tear Glands)	Slight secretion	Copious tear secretion
Parotid Glands	Viscous secretion	Watery secretion
Submaxillary Glands	Slight, thick secretion	Profuse, enzyme-rich secretion
Gastric Glands	Reduced secretion	Increased acid and enzyme secretion
Pancreas	Decreased secretion	Increased enzyme and insulin secretion
Sweat Glands (Eccrine)	Profuse sweating (cholinergic mediation)	No effect
Apocrine Glands	Thick, odorous secretion	No effect
Heart: Myocardium	Increased heart rate and force of contraction	Decreased heart rate and contractility

Heart: Coronary Vessels	Dilation (β2), constriction (α) – context-dependent	Dilation
Lungs: Bronchi	Bronchodilation	Bronchoconstriction
Lungs: Bronchial Vessels	Mild vasoconstriction	Vasodilation
Intestine: Smooth Muscle (Motility)	Decreased peristalsis and tone	Increased peristalsis and tone
Intestine: Sphincters	Increased tone (constriction)	Relaxation
Liver	Glycogenolysis and glucose release	Glycogen synthesis
Gallbladder & Bile Ducts	Relaxation	Contraction
Kidney	Decreased urine output (via vasoconstriction)	No significant effect
Bladder: Detrusor Muscle	Relaxation	Contraction
Bladder: Trigone & Sphincter	Contraction	Relaxation
Penis	Ejaculation	Erection
Systemic Arterioles: Abdominal Organs	Vasoconstriction	Minimal effect
Systemic Arterioles: Skeletal Muscle	Vasodilation (β2), vasoconstriction (α)	Minimal effect
Systemic Arterioles: Skin	Vasoconstriction	No effect

Blood: Coagulation	Increased clotting tendency	No direct effect
Blood: Glucose	Increased glucose (via glycogenolysis & gluconeogenesis)	Mild effect via insulin release
Blood: Lipids	Increased lipolysis	No direct effect
Basal Metabolism	Increased (up to 100%)	No significant effect
Adrenal Medulla	Secretion of adrenaline and noradrenaline	No effect
Mental Activity	Increased alertness	Relaxation, calmness
Piloerector Muscles	Contraction ("goosebumps")	No effect

Earth Sciences

Earth sciences are still
young people and they like it on Saturday nights
go dancing...
that's why progress is so slow

Francesco Salvi, 1998

Earth sciences have trudged along winding, uphill paths for centuries—sometimes millennia—while many of humanity's greatest discoveries have arrived by chance or through bursts of wild inspiration, like uninvited guests crashing the party of reason. In the dance between logic and intuition, it's often the untamed colt of human genius that leads the charge.

When the light of the intellect dims, the brilliance of the soul takes over—and the contrast is stark. One flickers like a weak bulb in a basement, while the other blazes like the noonday sun over a tropical sea.

The true secret of well-being may lie in our ability to exercise **free will**, to choose—consciously and courageously—how we shape our lives. Choosing what foods to allow into the temple of your body is no small matter. It's a foundational act of self-respect. Every conscious choice strengthens your inner resolve, shaping it into a laser beam of intent—one sharp enough to slice through even the thickest walls of bad habits.

So go forward, on purpose. Step boldly into your own metamorphosis, no matter where you are or who you're with. Be so tuned in to your values that you feel fully *at ease* refusing anti-orthomolecular junk food—whether you're at a neighborhood pizzeria or dining with the King of England who insists you honor his royal roast beef.

A helpful guideline to avoid becoming a joyless nutritional monk? Chase **pleasure**, not punishment. Enjoy the hell out of your alternative dishes. Don't sabotage your new path with mental landmines like:

"If I eat all those carrots, I'll turn into a rabbit!" "What am I, a cow? Look at all these vegetables!"

Smile. Laugh, even. Let joy coat every bite. Let your body rediscover what *well-being* actually tastes like.

Pain and suffering? Those are emotional cocktails—hormonal hurricanes stirred up in your brain. And like an experienced sailor, you have the tools to steer your ship through them. Decide **now** what empowering beliefs you want to plant into your life. And never forget: no pharmaceutical on Earth can compete with the potent healing compounds your own body produces—**if** you respect its balance and maintain its alkalinity.

In an alkaline environment, every organ and system thrives. They don't just function—they flourish. No one is forcing you to eat clean. But if you choose to indulge in low-vibration, inflammatory foods, don't act surprised when your health begins its slow slide into twilight.

Don't blame the doctors. Don't rage at the health system. Look inward. And if you made a Faustian bargain—trading your vitality and potential for a plate of porchetta and sausage—then own that choice. But know this: you can *always* make a new one.

NORMAL PH VALUES FOR ORGANS AND DISTRICTS

BLOOD 7.35-7.45

SALIVE 6.50-7.50

STOMACH 1.00-3.50

DUODENUM 4.80-8.20

FECES 4.60-8.40

URINE 4.50-8.40

LIVER BILE 7.10-8.50

GALLBALE 5.50-7.70

PANCREAS 8.00-8.30

(Scheme modified from Correlative Urinalysis by M.T. Morter,1987)

Panfhealing® is a fresh word for something ancient: the journey of reconnecting with your true self. We didn't invent it—because the real secret of healing is already within you. It's written in your cells, your breath, your intuition. And only you can decide when it's time to start that journey.

As Plato once said, *we don't really discover—we remember.* And that's what Panfhealing® and the pH@ Diet are about: remembering what the body already knows. They're not a trend or a hack—they're part of our human heritage. At the heart of it is one simple idea: your quality of life starts at the cellular level. That's where energy, joy, inflammation, stress, and disease begin—and where balance can be restored.

Here's why pH matters:

The acidity or alkalinity inside your body shapes the way your enzymes function. Enzymes influence the production of hormones and vitamins, which affect every cell, tissue, and organ in your body. It's all connected. The system is cyclical, delicate, and deeply intelligent.

Your body is designed to thrive in an alkaline state (ideally with a urinary pH around 6.5—more on that in the pH@ Diet, published by Tecniche Nuove). And while food and hydration are major players, your thoughts and emotions also shift your pH. A negative mindset, chronic stress, or toxic relationships can be more acidifying than a double cheeseburger.

Now, let's be real—your body won't just stop working if it's slightly acidic. But over time, that internal imbalance can slow everything down, drain your energy, weaken your immunity, and cloud your mental clarity. Staying alkaline isn't about perfection—it's about giving your body the conditions it needs to do what it does best: heal, regulate, and thrive.

What does this look like in practice? During Panfhealing® , you'll be encouraged to reduce acid-forming foods—think refined carbs, white bread and pasta, sugar, coffee, tea, processed sweets, and soda. Instead, load up on alkaline-forming foods like vegetables and fruit. Ideally, they should make up about 80% of your daily meals.

The more animal protein and processed food you consume, the more acidic your internal environment becomes—and the harder it is for your body to stay in balance. And yes, negative thoughts have a similar effect. Let's just say that an argument with your boss might be as acidifying as that rare steak you were trying to avoid.

Eating more plants isn't the only key—you also need to dial down protein intake to about 30 grams per day. That's roughly the size of a fast-food burger. One egg per day is the limit.

Think of it this way: would you walk into a sacred space—whether it's a meditation, a yoga class, or a spiritual ritual—after binging on fried meats and sugar? Probably not. That's why spiritual traditions across cultures often call for fasting or dietary purification before entering altered states. An alkaline body isn't just physically healthier—it's energetically lighter, clearer, and more attuned.

So when does acidity spike? Any time your body is under pressure. When you're in fight-or-flight mode—running on stress, sleep-deprived, overworked—your system starts burning through resources just to keep you going. Digestion slows. Recovery gets delayed. Acidic byproducts start building up. Your body isn't broken—it's just in survival mode.

Panfhealing® is your invitation to shift from survival to alignment. To support your body, your mind, and your inner life with every bite, breath, and thought.

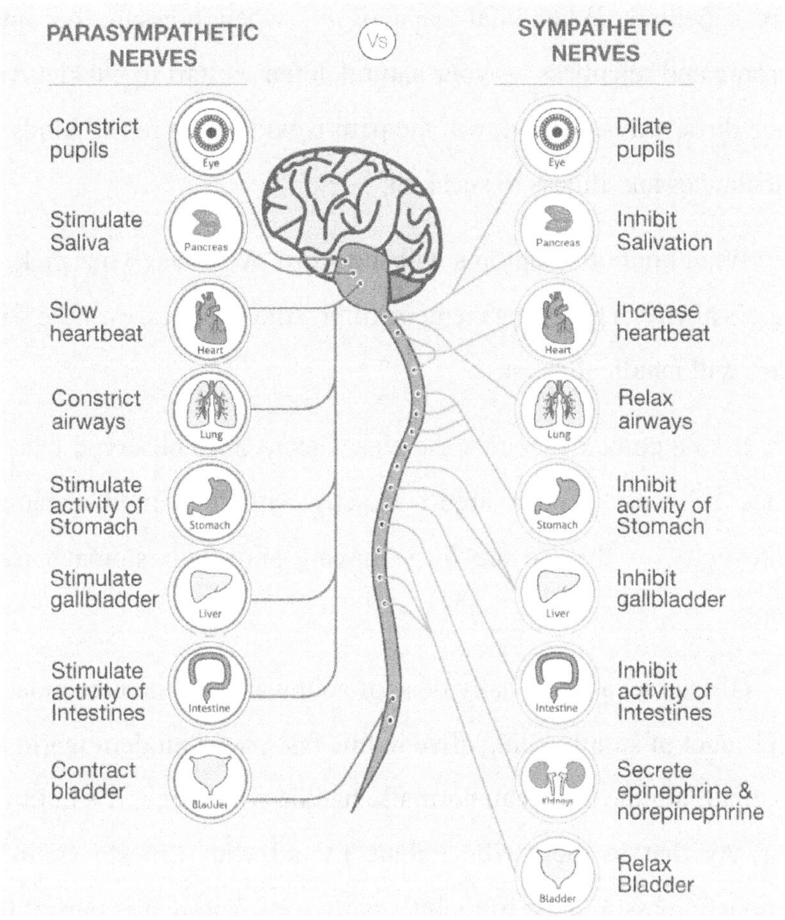

Just like in every marriage — no matter how blissful — there's always a meddling mother-in-law somewhere in the picture, stress and acidification are inseparable partners in crime: one doesn't show up without the other.

The real trouble begins when stress keeps knocking without giving the body enough time to clear out the excess acidic debris it leaves behind. When that happens — when pressure becomes chronic and relentless — your natural defenses start to buckle. And once those walls come down, the path is wide open for all kinds of imbalances and illness to sneak in.

What kind of symptoms will show up? Well, take your pick — there's always a generous menu on offer. And genetics, ever the wild card, will handle the rest.

It's no coincidence that the wise Cicero once observed that, in times of war, people aren't exactly sitting around debating philosophy — they're too busy making sure their stomach isn't empty.

Of course, a small daily dose of acid waste — the unavoidable byproduct of simply being alive in this fast-paced modern world — is something the body can normally handle with grace. It's built for that. As that iconic 1970s Italian TV ad with Ernesto Calindri famously reassured us: life's little daily wear-and-tear is part of the deal.

The real problem begins when those levels surge past the danger zone — when stress piles up faster than the body can clear it away. That's when the system flips into full-blown battle mode — every cell armed to the teeth, every resource diverted to the frontlines. And as anyone (especially Americans, who seem to have perfected the art of permanent warfare) can tell you: living in a constant state of emergency is wildly expensive, exhausting, and ultimately unsustainable.

The same is true for your inner army of cells. Mobilized for too long, without pause or peace, they begin to misfire. And from there, disturbances, dysfunctions, and diseases are never far behind.

Fortunately, science and research are now leading us right back to a wisdom we somehow forgot along the way: that the real art of living well — and long — lies not in fighting harder, but in learning how to prevent the battle in the first place.

And that begins with a return to nature. A return to balance. A return to care.

We Are Made Of The Same Material As Our Dreams

"Our souls travel through spaces of Life
not commensurable by the hourglass of time
invented by man to fence the sand of the ocean of the universe"

Panfhealing® personal communication

One can hardly argue with this statement often (perhaps wrongly) attributed to Shakespeare. After all, the human body is not a Sicilian cannoli stuffed with organs, nor is it a random collection of spare biochemical parts waiting to be replaced. No, the body is far more than an assembly line of receptors, cells, and organs. It's a living, breathing field of intelligent memory — constantly updating, communicating, and keeping every inch of you informed about what *was*, what *is*, and even what *might be*.

Many have tried — mostly in vain — to track down the "director" behind this dazzling, never-ending spectacle we call life. In fact, in the last century, some particularly enthusiastic scientists went so far as to *weigh* people moments before and moments after death, hoping to detect some measurable sign of the soul's departure. Spoiler: the experiment didn't exactly prove much — except maybe that if the soul exists, it's blessedly weightless.

And yet, consider this: with every single breath, you inhale and exhale around 10^{22} atoms — particles that may once have belonged to anyone or anything: Cleopatra, Einstein, Trump (for better or worse), or even the first fish that ever crawled onto land. Radioactive isotope studies have shown that — at the atomic level — we are all quietly sharing ourselves with the entire world.

In fact, over 98% of the atoms in your body right now will be gone and replaced within a single year.

→ Your stomach lining? Completely renewed in 5 days.
→ Your skin? Brand new in about a month.
→ Your liver? Rebuilt in 6 weeks.
→ Your skeleton? Refreshed in roughly 3 months.
→ Even your DNA? Its double helix strands get a full makeover every 6 weeks.

Not bad, right?

Which means — and let's just say it out loud — by the time you finish reading this book, you are *literally* not the same person who started it.

In a year? You'll be a completely new man or woman, from the first to the last atom — with only one thing holding all those particles together: your soul. The original organizing principle. The mysterious gravity that makes *you*...well, *you*.

In a strange way, you are living proof of life after death — because every second, some version of you dies…and yet, here you still are.

And maybe — just maybe — we *are* made of the same stuff as dreams.

Little fragments of fallen stars…desperately trying to return to the great ocean of energy from which, for reasons we still don't understand, we once emerged.

Panfhealing® Action Sites

Sources of Free Radicals

- NEGATIVE THOUGHTS (hatred, resentment, anger, revenge, anxiety, envy, pride)
- DIETARY ERRORS (excess protein, sweets, refined foods, alcohol, etc.)
- POLLUTION (magnetic fields, environmental toxins, UV radiation)
- LACK OF HYDRATION
- INADEQUATE OR EXCESSIVE PHYSICAL EXERCISE
- POOR SLEEP QUALITY
- LOW AIR QUALITY
- DRUGS

↓

Formation of Free Radicals → Damage to Lipids, Proteins, and Nucleic Acids (DNA, RNA)

↓

Degeneration of Cellular Functions

↓

Aging

↓

Development of Diseases That Benefit from Reducing Free Radicals

Modern medicine, often focused merely on the treatment of symptoms, is gradually giving way to new and exciting paradigms — broader, unifying models that no longer criminalize the presence of disease, but rather seek to understand its meaning within a larger context. These models bring together seemingly unrelated disorders under a single, vast category: pathologies linked to oxidative stress and free radicals.

Among them:

- Cancer
- Cardiovascular diseases
- Asthma
- Emphysema
- Rheumatoid arthritis
- Cataracts
- Heart attack
- Obesity
- Colitis

- Diabetes
- Ulcers
- Ulcerative colitis
- Crohn's disease
- Autoimmune diseases
- Mental health disorders
- Osteoporosis
- Arteriosclerosis

Just as rust corrodes metal, a lack of oxygen can gradually deteriorate the life quality of our cells.

The acquisition of new and essential scientific insights into the biochemistry of cellular oxidation has revealed how the selective permeability of cell membranes can be altered, triggering symptoms and diseases in various organs and systems. And yet, at the root of it all, the common denominator remains: oxygen deficiency.

Diabetes, heart attacks, strokes, or cancer may present diverse clinical pictures — but fundamentally, they arise from the same cause: the poor efficiency of the body's antioxidant defences.

Today, over 1,000 potentially oncogenic chemical substances have been identified. But beyond chemicals, other factors — ionizing and ultraviolet radiation, certain types of dental amalgams (gamma 1 and gamma 2), and some viruses — can also disrupt cellular metabolic balance.

And here lies a crucial observation: the cancer cell is not, in fact, an insane or anarchic entity. On the contrary — as Warburg rightly pointed out — it is a highly adaptive cell, capable of extraordinary flexibility in the face of oxygen deficiency. What we call a neoplastic cell is nothing more than a normal cell forced to "tighten its belt" in order to survive in a hostile environment.

As early as 1960, Louis Claude Vincent demonstrated the role played by the individual biological terrain as a predisposing factor in the onset of major diseases, including cancer. This scientist — now somewhat forgotten — had already grasped the simple and clear mechanism underlying these pathologies. He was even officially commissioned by the French Ministry of Health to investigate why certain French cities experienced higher mortality rates than others.

Vincent's findings confirmed that an alkaline-oxidized organism, deprived of electrons and oxygen, represented the ideal breeding ground for cancer. In these environments, the growth of common yeasts such as *Candida albicans* would be favored — consistent with the Fermentation Theory — leading to an excessive production of lactate due to reduced efficiency of the Tricarboxylic Acid Cycle.

In essence: without oxygen, one either dies immediately or slowly. If you stop breathing, the truth is immediate. But if cellular and mitochondrial respiration is interrupted through erroneous lifestyle and behavioral patterns, the alarm bells are often silent — until neoplastic cells emerge as a survival strategy.

Non-invasive, cost-effective, and innovative methods such as BEV (Bioelectronics of Vincent) and BTA (Biological Terrain Analysis) now make it possible to assess general oxidative stress across various regions of the body. These tools offer a chance to intervene well before damage to specific organs becomes irreversible.

Free radicals target cellular proteins as a primary objective, denaturing them and altering their functions. Their insatiable hunger for electrons — essential fuel for the mitochondria, the energy powerhouses of cells — is particularly damaging.

Even the loss of a single electron in the delicate metabolic balance of the organism can trigger disastrous consequences, setting off chain reactions that render a molecule biologically useless or even harmful.

Some free radicals can even link two molecules together, creating a rigid, inert compound called an *aldehyde*. When these accumulate in visco-elastic structures — tendons, muscles, or collagen — they lead to deterioration, stiffening, and, ultimately, premature aging.

Existential Conflicts With Parents

You are free before the sun of the day,

You are free before the stars of the night;

And you are free when there is no sun, no moon, no stars.

You are free even when you close your eyes to all things.

But you are a slave to the person who loves you, because he loves you.

Kahlil Gibran from "Sand and Foam"

In the Hindu epic *Mahabharata*, the mythical warrior Arjuna, when describing the art of falcon hunting, conveys through his stance the idea of composure and inner peace. In that moment, he is the man whose consciousness has been awakened, who knows neither anger nor fear (lucky him!), and remains unshaken by adversity.

Often, great fortune arises from loss, and defeat is borne from excess, as can be deduced from a reading of the *Tao Te Ching*. Therefore, maintaining balance is a fundamental requirement for living in harmony with oneself and the universe. Raising a child, for instance, is no small task, and this commitment cannot be undertaken without the inner resources necessary to pass on to this soul who will share precious moments with us as they form their path.

Education that aims only to transmit working or behavioral techniques (whether religious, moral, or otherwise), which are already part of a social group's heritage and aimed at maintaining their relative immutability, can be carried out with the mere technical discipline of impersonal teaching. On the other hand, the aspiration to not only transmit these acquired didactic structures but to also enable individuals to perfect these techniques and forge their own destinies is an entirely different endeavor.

In offspring, the imprinting mechanism is innate (from the English "impression"), a modeling process based on the ability to identify with the behavior of others. No mammal or vertebrate is born able to adequately discern external objects, undergoing this conditioning process to develop an irreversible attachment. This imprinting period is shorter the less evolved the species in question is. Between a chick and a hen, this bond lasts anywhere from a few hours to a few days, while in humans, it can persist for significantly longer periods, and even extend to one's habitat (Habitat Imprinting), food, and sexual preferences (Food Imprinting and Sexual Imprinting).

The closest imprinting models, from a spatio-temporal perspective, for a newborn will first and foremost be human beings of the same species—the mother, then the father, the grandmother, the babysitter, etc., depending on the social-familial organization. A mother who entrusts her child to a nanny because she's overly consumed by her managerial career rather than by her new responsibilities as a mother, risks seeing the role of reference model usurped by the caregiver, as the filial imprinting gets hijacked toward someone physically present.

A child spontaneously elects, in the first years of life (especially the first three), which human figure to distill what we call "teachings." For this process to occur, the child will rely on the simple rules of physical presence and the willingness for playful contact demonstrated by the human figure who enters into pedagogical symbiosis with them.

In adulthood, the imprinted object becomes the recipient of social and sexual behaviors, and it can thus be deduced that it plays a crucial role in identifying one's own species.

Many modern families place a disproportionate emphasis on enrolling their newborns in specialized, expensive, flashy institutions—a behavior even more foreign to our less evolved primate cousins. The importance of one's offspring's growth is a requirement that demands the physical presence of the mother.

Female orangutans display more maternal behaviors than many human mothers we encounter throughout our lives. They don't seem inclined to turn to outside structures for raising their young...

To an external observer, this behavior may seem absurd, even incoherent, and thus the question becomes legitimate:

"Why bother having a child if you're just going to send them off to daycare a few months later? Should we attend monkey school?"

Well, that wouldn't be such a bad idea, assuming there are any primates willing to do it after the regrettable Tarzan episode...

A gynecologist friend of mine cynically argued that this habit of easily parking children might reflect the search for simple erotic gratification through the act of completing a sexual relationship nine months before birth—without true awareness of the couple's role in the act—which only serves to perpetuate the species according to Spencer's theories.

Certainly, an unwanted child can become a great burden for parents, and such conflicting messages often travel faster than the Italian postal service, right into the heart of this innocent creature, shaping its development, growth, and life.

To exorcise any guilt over the new "tenant's" default, the parent-hoteliers will gladly pay a financial price to guarantee a healthy and constructive education for the child. Not bad for busy parents! They've managed to establish, right from the beginning, a relationship with an exquisite hotel flavor, where the rhythms blend harmoniously with the needs and schedules of the spouses.

Everything runs like a Swiss watch: the child is picked up by the nursery school bus at 8:00 AM, returned at 4:00 PM, already fed, changed, and entertained, ready to be placed in front of the TV to watch "The Sword in the Stone" or "Pocahontas" until at least 6:30 PM. Then, it's time for another good hour with the other two tenants (Father and Mother) in the company of the evening news or a satirical TV show, where the usual interviewer is kicked by the politician who doesn't want to be interviewed!

And then one day, when this child grows up, they'll rightfully be able to call Oprah Winfrey or Kelly Clarkson "mom"… and if they stay up late one evening... well, in this case, they'll find Jimmy Fallon as their foster dad.

Beyond the paradoxical chill of this metaphor of industrialization, take note: at least someone is dedicating their evenings to nurturing human values, which characters in search of authorship, like your children, will one day reference—like David Letterman, who has tirelessly professed from the Ed Sullivan Theatre in NY for years.

Kaizen:

Constant Improvement

Challenges mobilize resources,

They raise awareness,

They sharpen the senses....

Koan Zen

The Tao teaches us that life flows like a torrent — powerful, unstoppable, and alive. The wise person, like water, moves with fluid grace but with unshakable strength, always finding a way forward, overcoming obstacles, just as mountain streams carve their way uphill against all odds.

To live, for every living being, is to embrace change — a continuous process of mutation and transformation within the eternal cycles of creation.

The true healer, in this view, is not the one who selects only easy cases or perfect patients, but the one who welcomes every soul. A true healer acts as a catalyst for growth — facilitating the evolution of those who, through suffering, are awakening to new levels of awareness.

Standing on the shoulders of those who came before us is the foundation of all great knowledge. In science, every discovery is built upon previous insights.

The Japanese even coined a word for this principle: *Kaizen* — meaning continuous improvement. It speaks to the wisdom of learning from the past in order to generate steady, incremental growth, day after day.

A staircase is made of many steps — each one essential, none less important than the other — all contributing to the journey toward higher understanding or success.

Every great inventor has drawn inspiration from the work of others. Just as every child learns by imitating the world around them, growth is built on models, on example, on connection.

You, in every action and every word, are shaping the inner world of another human being. The behaviors they adopt, the choices they make, will often be a direct reflection of their emotional landscape — a landscape shaped, in part, by the models and values you have transmitted with love and consistency.

Your values will define the direction of your life — and through you, the lives of your children and those around you. This is why it is so essential to understand your *true* values — because clarity in this area will allow you to live in deeper alignment with your aspirations, and to experience a more authentic, sustained happiness. When you commit to living according to your core values — rather than chasing superficial goals — you cultivate a sense of deep fulfillment. And from this place of integrity and joy, those around you will naturally draw strength, warmth, and love.

Think of life as a long and beautiful journey along an infinite path. And perhaps the greatest risk along this path is not failure — but losing your balance. This is why Taoist sages have always emphasized the principle of *Zhong* — the art of balance, moderation, and centeredness.

Now it's your turn. Take a pen and a blank sheet of paper.

On the left side, write down what you believe to be your goal values — the things that give your life meaning and purpose.

On the right side, write your instrumental values — the tools, behaviors, and attitudes that can help you move closer to those goals.

Yes — right now. Give yourself 10 minutes. Be honest. Write without hesitation. And above all — write with sincerity.

The Dentist Of The Gold Prosthesis

Eurystheus, having observed how Hercules achieved control of the mind
and led the bull of desire into the temple of the soul
like a gentle lamb in the fold,
he decided to entrust him with the task of conquering the golden apples in the garden of the Hesperides.

The Path of Discipleship Through the Zodiac – Alice A. Bailey

I once knew a dentist who had grown up in dignified poverty — a kind of hardship softened only by the tireless sacrifices of his family, who somehow managed to support him through all his years of study.

Not a day passed without him swearing to himself — and to the heavens — that he would change his fate at any cost. Yet in doing so, he grew increasingly ashamed of his humble origins, distancing himself from the very family whose love had carried him that far.

He was intelligent, yes — but also deeply ambitious and painfully insecure. This toxic mix made him cunning rather than wise, and willing to strike a deal with any passing Faust if it promised him power or wealth.

In time, he became both rich and famous. In his city, he was known as *The Dentist of the Golden Prostheses* — not only for the literal gold in his dental work, but even more so for the exorbitant prices he charged.

For him, money became the ultimate proof of skill. The more he earned, the more he craved — money and recognition feeding each other in a perfect storm of insatiable appetite. No day went by without him proposing costly, sophisticated prosthetic procedures — often well beyond the financial reach of his patients, who, dazzled by his charisma and persuasion, frequently gave in.

His obsession with wealth devoured everything else. He neglected his wife. He neglected his son. He pursued only his career, convinced that money could patch the wounds of a childhood shaped by scarcity — a childhood where his father's meager laborer's salary barely stretched to cover essentials, let alone dreams.

He told himself that luxury was medicine — fast cars, expensive watches, designer suits, glamorous women drawn not to *him* but to the glittering aura he projected.

And for a time, it seemed to work. Until, one grey February afternoon, Faust himself arrived — punctual as ever — to collect what was owed.

You see, Faust is generous when he lends. But when it's time to settle accounts, he is neither forgetful nor forgiving.

Yet even in the dark recesses of that ancient pact, there remains one slim loophole: redemption. If, at some point, the debtor has performed a single, selfless act — an unprofitable gesture born of pure humanity — then the debt might just be forgiven.

The dentist might have escaped. *Might*.

That day, Faust came disguised as an elderly man — poor, disheveled, suffering visibly from a raging dental abscess. In a low voice, he admitted he had no money to pay. A test, plain as day.

But the dentist, blind in his greed, saw only a worthless patient wasting his time. Furious, he threw him out, cursing him back to the streets.

That old man — that discarded patient — was Faust himself.

And when night fell, and the golden dental chair was once again occupied by another wealthy client, Faust's shadow had already begun to loom large behind him.

But setting aside that unfortunate encounter with Faust — who, as we know, always keeps score — one night the cynical dentist came home even later than usual. And for him, *usual* was already scandalously late. In fact, it was practically morning.

He had just spent yet another night in the company of some glamorous woman — and judging by his unsteady steps and glassy eyes, he hadn't exactly stuck to mineral water.

But this time, something was different.

Waiting for him at home wasn't his long-suffering wife — not her, not her exhausted silence, not even her usual resigned tears. No, waiting for him was a simple note. Short. Surgical. Almost clinical in tone.

She had left him. Forever. And, adding insult to injury, she hadn't run off with just anyone — but with a certain well-known banker named Faust.

Oh, the irony.

Apparently, the desperate wife — worn down by years of loneliness, humiliation, and those shirts reeking of perfume and stained with lipstick (which she, like some tragic laundress of lost love, washed over and over in vain) — had finally decided to cash in her own revenge.

And her own Faust had been only too happy to oblige.

As if that weren't enough, a few months earlier, his only son, Paolo — the same Paolo he had barely noticed growing up — had fallen hard into drugs. Not medical school, as his father had so pompously dreamed. Not dentistry, God forbid. No, Paolo had ended up in a commune somewhere, trying to detox, trying maybe just to breathe air that wasn't poisoned by money, status, or resentment.

The illustrious father, now newly minted as a professor at some little-known university, naturally had no time to visit him. Busy, always busy. And, deep down, ashamed.

Ashamed just like he had once been of his own poor parents.

A professor with a junkie son — hardly the kind of detail you wanted in your elegant professional résumé.

Better to bury that little scandal like a stone in the ground. Out of sight, out of mind.

And so this was the bitter epilogue of a story that had begun in hunger and ended in excess — a story not particularly cheerful, not particularly original, but brutally effective all the same.

The once-rampant doctor was now utterly, spectacularly alone.

Sure, his bank account was still thriving — fat, muscular, and obscene.

But it turns out that even the fattest bank account can't buy you immunity from certain forms of cosmic justice.

And his arrived right on time, in the form of a crushing, suffocating depression — the kind no money in the world can anesthetize.

This story, of course, isn't meant to cast judgment on the medical profession, much less on dentists — most of whom would hardly recognize themselves in a character like this. For obvious reasons of discretion, we won't reveal any further identifying details.

But what's clear is that this man's choice to chase after *instrumental* values — things like money, status, and appearances — rather than true, *essential* values made him easy prey to his own greed.

And so, the moral of this little metaphor practically shouts at us: money is a tool, never a destination.

If you decide to worship at the altar of wealth — if you mistake it for life's ultimate goal — you'll soon discover that suffering is part of the bargain. Because sooner or later, waiting around some unexpected corner, there's always a Doctor Faust ready to collect.

That painful lesson came crashing down on the doctor's life with merciless force. He learned it — maybe too late — through the double, searing loss of his son first, and then his wife.

His son, Paolo, had grown up starved for guidance, deprived of any real emotional compass. And so, like many lost children, he sought refuge in the only escape hatch he could find — drugs. His father, a distant, distracted presence at best, had failed to offer him the one thing a parent must always give: a sense of worth rooted in love, not achievement.

Getting clean is never easy. Paolo tried. He ended up in a commune, surrounded by people who genuinely cared. But the absence of his father — or maybe simply the absence of feeling truly loved — left a wound no detox could reach.

Sick, tired, and HIV-positive, Paolo couldn't go on. And one summer evening, while his father, the wealthy dentist, was lounging aboard a yacht in Sardinia — playing at being a king in some hollow paradise — Paolo ended his life.

And so the wheel turned.

His wife, meanwhile, rebuilt her life with another man — yes, the same Doctor Faust — and that glittering mirage of success the dentist had once chased crumbled like dust when Faust eventually demanded his price.

Today, that same dentist works as a volunteer missionary in Southern Africa. Maybe — God willing — he has finally found some measure of peace, tending to the suffering of others in a way he never managed with those closest to him. There, far from yachts and stained shirts and empty victories, he offers his skills for free to those who need them most.

And maybe, for the first time in his life, he's truly healing someone — including himself.

Being a parent is no easy task, as Kahlil Gibran's poem so sweetly suggests. Perhaps you'll feel compelled to copy it down by hand, or perhaps, if someone you've loved is no longer with you, you'll send it to the address where you imagine they still dwell. It doesn't matter if the address is unreachable by ordinary means — trust that the letter will still arrive, even if the journey is beyond the bounds of reason.

For the postal service used here is the most reliable of all: the one that never goes on strike, the one that always delivers — even beyond the limits of what we know.

Here is what the poet says:

And a woman who had a child at her breast said:
Tell us about the children.
And he said:

Your children are not your children,
but they are the sons and daughters of the desire that life brings within itself.
They do not come from you, but through you,
and although they live with you, they do not belong to you.

You can give them your love, but not your thoughts,
for they have their own thoughts.
You may house their bodies, but not their souls,
for these live in the house of tomorrow,
which you cannot visit, not even in a dream.

You can strive to be like them,
but do not try to make them like you.
For life does not go backwards, nor does it waste time with yesterday.
You are the bows from which your children are shot,
like living arrows.
The Archer sees clearly the target on the path of infinity,
and with his strength he bends you so that his arrows go far and fast.

Let the Archer's hand be joyfully extended,
for if he loves the flying arrow, he loves the solid bow equally.

This wisdom is not just about love, but about the monumental challenge of parenting — and, perhaps most importantly, the understanding that our children are not ours to shape, but rather to guide. They arrive with their own souls, their own destinies, their own arrows already drawn.

The true lesson for us as parents lies in recognizing this profound responsibility — to guide, to love, but not to control. To *allow* them to unfold into their own beings.

The path to healing begins here: understanding that as much as we long to protect them, our role is to prepare them to find their own strength, even if it means they will sometimes fall or stray from the path.

This realization doesn't come easily. Many of the hardest emotions we will face as parents are born from this very struggle. The pain of seeing a child suffer or fail, the fear of not doing enough, the heartbreak of watching them struggle with their own battles — these are the most difficult wounds to heal.

But, as we accept the gift of these relationships, and the inevitability of their impermanence, we begin to see that in the end, it is not what we do for them, but what we allow them to do for themselves, that will shape their journey.

We don't have a recipe for raising children, nor can we pretend to have one. But we can offer this simple guidance: live according to your highest ideals. Be true to the meaning you've found in your life. And, above all, trust that the same God who resides in us all will guide them, just as He guides us.

The most challenging emotions to overcome are often those tied to our loved ones, especially in the sacred bond between parent and child. When these emotions arise, remember this: the struggles we face are part of the deeper, often painful, work of education. We help shape them not by forcing them into our image, but by letting them rise in their own.

The most common negative emotion that surfaced during the Panfhealing® stages was the fear of being rejected by those we love or by the social and family circles we belong to — much like what happened to the dentist's son. Anger toward a parent can stem from the feeling that they don't know what matters most to you, and, perhaps unwittingly, have broken values that are significant to you and have caused you pain. If you've suffered in this way, try to remember that, in the end, they do love you. Imagine holding them tenderly, as though they were your children and you their parent... yes, we're suggesting a role reversal. Picture a time when they won't be there with you because nature's biological law will take them away, and you'll miss them forever. When you think of them with longing and regret, that bitterness in your heart will vanish as quickly as morning mist lifts under the noon sun.

Here's a chance for you to seize: forgive now, for tomorrow may be too late. If forgiveness isn't part of your plans today, keep in mind that your rules might be wrong, even if you hold them as strict and infallible. Over time, life's perspectives shift — often unexpectedly — and what once seemed like the ultimate goal of your desires may lose its meaning entirely, no longer stirring even the faintest trace of interest in you.

As you journey through life, you may find yourself looking at a distant landscape, imagining its beauty, but as you get closer, it turns out to be completely different from what you envisioned. Life often changes our goals, because, as the traveler moves forward, they change. By the time you arrive at your destination, you may not be the same person who set out.

Being flexible, open to change, and adaptable will help you find happiness and serenity. Happiness does not depend on what you acquire, but on the awareness of who you truly are. I have seen patients with only one lung breathe freely, the limping and the lame walk with confidence, the blind experience the light, the severely burned feel beautiful and graceful, and the obese glide weightlessly like a hippopotamus in Walt Disney's *Fantasia* — all grateful for the half-full glass life has allowed them to savor. And yet, I've seen people with perfect bodies, living according to society's standards of beauty, feel wretched and repulsive. I've witnessed undefeated champions collapse exhausted on the stairs at home.

Happiness is not about what you possess, but about how you understand and accept yourself.

With Panfhealing®, you can heal from these situations by learning the transformative power of self-forgiveness. This process increases your awareness, helping you let go of the tendency to judge others, which, when directed toward your parents, can become a dangerous boomerang. Every time you judge someone, you're placing yourself — not the person being judged — in a cage. Judgment does not define the other, but you.

You will come to accept that others are entitled to walk their own paths, different from yours, yet no less valid or true. Let others direct their lives, and instead of trying to control them, sit back as a spectator and applaud. You will learn to see others for who they truly are, not for who you wish them to be. In doing so, you'll give both yourself and others more room to breathe, embracing aspects you once found irritating or frustrating. As Carl Jung wisely said, "Everything that irritates us in others can lead us to understand ourselves."

Letting go of one's illusory ego means untangling the maze of conflicts it has built. As Tagore deeply reflects in one of his meditations, the ego is like a wall that traps the human spirit in the dungeons of frustration:

He whom I invoke by my name despairs in these prisons.
I'm so consumed by enclosing myself within this wall,
which grows taller by the moment,
that I lose sight of my true self in its dark shadow.
Yet, I am delighted with this immense wall I tirelessly construct
from sand and dust,
making sure not a single flaw can destabilize it.
I work so hard and so meticulously
that I forget my true essence.

This capricious ego lives off illusions, feeding you the belief in separateness. In those moments when you feel alone, abandoned, isolated, it tightens its grip around your neck like iron pincers. A classic cartoon character who embodies these traits is the unforgettable Scrooge McDuck. With his obsessive drive to amass wealth, he lives alone in his warehouse, wallowing in his private ocean of endless gold coins, locked away from the world.

The seed of this separation is planted early. A newborn smiles naturally at anyone who comes near, offering pure, unguarded joy without expectation, simply because they exist in the serene awareness of unity. But it is you, the parents, who first begin to introduce the "give-and-take" of modern civilization, subtly interrupting the child's bliss. Phrases like "Eat your baby food for Daddy," or "If you don't do this, Mommy will cry," or "Be a good boy, or Daddy and Mommy will be angry," begin to seed the child with the notion that love and approval are conditional.

As the child grows, so does their experience of loneliness, criticism, and isolation, shaping their sense of separateness from their true self. They come to believe that physical life is everything, and they begin to devise strategies to be better than others, to extract the best from anyone they encounter.

Then, when the darkest tolls of life's bell ring, moments of bitter demotivation may flood in. The lack of existential purpose will clash with the overwhelming, iron-clad belief that life's path is a cycle of birth, suffering, and death — a cycle inescapable, where one must fight for everything they want, battling others in the process. The ego convinces them that acquiring more will bring peace, so they seek external validation, tackling their struggles the wrong way.

The truth, however, is that possession will never bring the peace or fulfillment their soul, imprisoned in Tagore's metaphorical dungeon, so desperately craves. Panfhealing® acts like a mighty force, detonating the old ego, shattering its constraints, and bringing the true self to the surface. It helps you recognize your true spiritual identity, guiding you through the profound journey into your inner sanctuary, where everything is one and inseparable.

The Thaumaturgic Power Of Forgiveness

The look of things varies
According to emotions,
And so we see magic and beauty in them:
But beauty and magic are actually in us

Kahlil Gibran - The Broken Wings

Feeling is the fuel of any healing journey — and the ultimate healing act is forgiveness. Only those who forgive can, in turn, be forgiven. It almost seems to sanction a kind of cosmic imperative.

Without the catalytic power of forgiveness — an extreme act of love — medicine risks becoming little more than tissue manipulation, a chemical procedure dressed up as care.

In fact, turning the other cheek to one's enemy produces countless benefits for the forgiver — far more, in most cases, than for the forgiven. The healing power of forgiveness is immense. It will allow you to uncover lessons during your Panfhealing® sessions that will leave you grateful to yourself — because, in your truest self, you will find the master or sage you've been seeking all along.

Avoid harsh judgment. Practice forgiveness. These are the true recipes for inner and physical well-being. Serenity will flow abundantly into your life, drawing positive people, fortunate events, happiness, and prosperity your way — because the cosmic law that "like attracts like" never fails.

Forgiveness, quite simply, works. And it's far more alkalizing than a pound of baking soda.

Quoting Christ may be unfashionable these days — but we'll never tire of doing it. His life and his message (not only the canonical parts) offer timeless light and healing, a balm for body and soul. Properly understood, they may even hold the keys to healing the world.

As Jesus told his disciples in the Gospel of Luke (17:3-4):

"If your brother sins, rebuke him; and if he repents, forgive him. And if he sins against you seven times in a day, and seven times comes back to you saying, 'I repent,' you must forgive him."

Nearly two thousand years have passed since the Son of Man came to teach humanity the Way, the Truth, and the Life. Simply by offering health to the sick, wisdom to the ignorant, and joy to the poor, he set off an earthquake in the political landscape of his time

— the tremors of which still register on the seismographs of human consciousness today.

His words remain vibrantly alive, unmatched in power, even if diluted, twisted, or distorted by those who came after. Sadly, as with many essential truths, the moment human hands begin to meddle, we see the classic "Telephone Game" effect: everyone reshaping the message to fit their own agenda, exploiting it, debasing it, stripping it of its original force.

The Aramaic Manuscript of the Essene Gospel of Peace (E.B. Szekely, 1937) is said to be kept in the Secret Archives of the Vatican, while the Slavonic Manuscript rests in the Royal Archives of the Habsburgs, now property of the Austrian government. The survival of these texts is due to Nestorian priests who, fleeing the advance of Genghis Khan's armies, took refuge in the West, carrying with them their icons and manuscripts.

Reading these documents offers a startling sense of truth — truths humanity, more than ever, deserves to reclaim in their fullness and integrity.

Sifting through these foundational texts — which shaped the religion of half the planet — will be an urgent task for the Church, understood as a human, temporal institution, if it hopes to survive in an age of rapid and radical change.

Historic events like the burning of the Library of Alexandria, or the decisions made by bishops and prelates at Councils like Nicaea (325), Constantinople (381), Ephesus (431), or the Synod of 531, have politically manipulated and substantially altered the contents and concepts of Christ's original Word.

Rediscovering the authentic exegetical sources of this universal, Christic message of love could help form better human beings — and better doctors — who treat their patients not just with pharmaceuticals, but with the most powerful medicine of all: the medicine of the heart — Forgiveness.

Throw a boomerang of love if you want love to return to you. This is the advice for the next millennium — a path to grace and self-sufficiency that aligns you directly with God and with the universal truths of which we are all participants and witnesses.

Remember: you can only truly harm others if you are sick yourself. Clinging to hatred for those who have hurt you will not heal you. On the contrary — it will bind you to them in a toxic chain of resentment, dragging you deeper into the abyss of negative, acidifying emotions.

A simple, powerful nightly practice to detox your soul and set yourself free.

"Don't be afraid to turn hate into love. It won't make you weak. It won't make you look like a loser. In fact, it might just be the greatest victory of your life."

Every night before going to sleep, give yourself a gift: A few quiet moments. A few deep breaths. And the courage to let go.

Close your eyes. Visualize the face of someone you resent — gently, without judgment — and invite them into the safe space of your inner sanctuary. Then, with calm and conviction, speak these words aloud:

THE THREE-STAGE FORMULA OF FORGIVENESS

(to be spoken out loud, ideally before bedtime)

1. **Forgive those who hurt you:**

    "I forgive you for whatever you did to me."

2. Forgive on behalf of life itself:

    "I forgive you too, even if you're not here with me right now."

3. **Forgive yourself:**

"I forgive myself for having suffered because of this resentment."

Why is self-forgiveness the most powerful of all?

Because holding on to resentment is like drinking poison and expecting someone else to get sick. And forgiveness is not weakness— it's inner detox. It's spiritual hygiene.

Forgiveness has been at the heart of healing rituals for millennia— from the Christian tradition of confession and Eucharist, to the Buddhist practice of compassion. It's time for modern preventive medicine to reclaim its power too.

This simple ritual, practiced consistently, can have a deeply calming, alkalizing effect on body and mind — like clearing the clogged pipes of your consciousness with a cosmic Liquid-Plumr.

Will it change the person who hurt you? Probably not.

But it *will* change you.

And that's where true healing begins.

Negative thoughts are not like parking tickets — you *can* return them to sender. Picture them stamped: *Recipient Unknown*. Then watch them dissolve into the great sea of cosmic nothingness, where all things forgotten eventually go.

Try it tonight. What's the worst that could happen? More peace? More freedom? Sounds like a win.

For You Who Suffer

When I sowed the seed of my pain
In the never plowed field of patience,
the sprout of faith has blossomed
and I gathered the fruit of happiness.

Speech - IDM turin

Don't be afraid to turn hate into love. It won't make you look weak — it'll make you victorious. Because the real battle isn't out there — it's in here. And when you win that battle, nothing and no one owns you anymore.

Every night, before sleep pulls you under, give yourself a moment. Breathe deep. Feel your chest soften. Then, summon — calmly, clearly — the person who hurt you. Bring them into your inner sanctuary, like a ghost at peace with being seen. And when they stand there, in your mind's quiet temple, say these words out loud — with conviction that cuts through bone.

THE THREE-STEP FORMULA OF FORGIVENESS

(From the PANFHEALING® method — a ritual for radical peace)

STEP 1: Forgive Those Who Hurt You.

"I forgive you for whatever you did to me."

No conditions. No ifs. No buts.

STEP 2: Forgive on Behalf of Others.

"I forgive you too, even though you're not here. Even though you'll never ask for it."

This isn't about them. It's about you unhooking the chain.

STEP 3: Forgive Yourself.

"I forgive my life for accepting to suffer because of this resentment."

This is the real revolution. This is where healing lives.

Note: Self-forgiveness is the nuclear core of this process — especially if your body's been carrying the slow poison of resentment for years. Heart disease. Tumors. Autoimmune flare-ups. Chronic pain. The body listens to every word the heart refuses to say.

Every wisdom tradition knew it: Christian confession, Buddhist compassion — these aren't just spiritual practices; they're ancient detox systems for the soul. Preventive medicine is only now catching up.

Say this Formula before bed. Every night. With your heart wide open. It costs nothing. But it pays in peace.

Forgiveness is the ultimate alkalizer. It's Liquid-Plumr for the pipes of your conscience — unclogging bitterness, flushing hate, restoring flow. It doesn't change the past. It changes you — and that's where reality begins to shift.

Try it. Test it like a scientist of the soul. Watch what happens.

THE COSMIC RULEBOOK THEY DON'T TEACH IN SCHOOL

The mind is small. The Absolute is not. And the tiny human brain — brilliant as it may be — doesn't have the software to decode infinity.

We can't see the whole pattern because we *are* the pattern. Pieces in a game older than time. Climbers on a golden staircase of awareness — where every step up costs sweat, pain, maybe tears.

Suffering is the shadow twin of pleasure. You don't get one without the other. And the higher you climb, the more solitary the journey becomes. Not lonely — just stripped down. You. Your courage. Your heart versus the hard truths of life.

Nothing in your story is random. Not love. Not loss. Not pain. Everything obeys the ancient law of cause and effect. Call it Karma. Call it Physics. Same thing.

And while the mind gropes in the dark, the heart sorts what's real from what's noise. Pain doesn't always harm. Pleasure doesn't always heal. Sometimes the thing that broke you was saving you from something worse.

WHEN YOU LOSE SOMEONE — LET THEM GO LIKE A WARRIOR

If grief has wrecked you — if you've lost someone who mattered like breath — remember this:

The soul isn't a prisoner of skin and bones. Death is not exile — it's homecoming. Bless their journey. Thank the universe for every second you shared. Then set them free.

Say goodbye — really say it.

Let your pain speak its message. Don't numb it. Don't drown it in pills or distractions.

Pain is information. A warning. A lesson dressed in thorns.

FOR YOU — YES, YOU — WHO HAVE KNOWN THE NIGHT

For you who sat shivering on a frozen sidewalk, wrapped in cardboard while the city lights never saw you.

For you in the streets of Chicago in December, too cold to even piss without freezing.

For you who once dreamed the Great American Dream… and woke up to the Great Nightmare dropped like napalm on another man's sky.

This forgiveness — this gritty, radical love — is for you most of all.

For you who donate blood to lower your blood pressure
but can't even say good morning to the office secretary.

For you who feel happier finishing your job than starting it.
For you who smile at those who broke you.
For you who bring flowers to someone who's lived through hell.

For you who pray in the silence of your heart.
For you who can only pray inside a church —
because your heart makes too much noise.

For you still dying today defending a religion
that never fed you
while your children starved.

For you who killed women and children in the name of that same God.
For you who sold weapons to the ones now waging war.

For you — model of discipline at work —
who clocks out and betrays wives, husbands, partners like clockwork.

For you who abort because condoms suck —
but never learned that by the third month
a baby can cry when torn from the womb.

For you who left a newborn in a dumpster
because you couldn't afford to feed him.
For you who rented a desperate woman's womb
when maybe digging through life's trash would've been enough.

For you who clone men to feel a little more like God.

For you who swear New York water is the best in the world.
For you who believed it.
For you whose kidneys have more calcium
than my washing machine filter.

For you who drink from PVC bottles
and then freak out about dioxin in Seveso (Italy) —
guess what PVC turns into when it breaks down?

For you who'd nail Christ even better this time —
because He came back.

For you who think your religion's better —
because it's yours.

For you waging holy wars.
For you believing that killing in war
is sacred.

For you who don't "do politics."
For you who do nothing else.
For you who steal anyway.

For you who drink cow's milk —
while cows never drink yours.

For you who believe it's true
because the news said so.

For you who read the obituaries —
hoping not to find your name there.

For you who glued your shoes to the wall.
For you who forgot your checkbook —
but protest like hell if they don't pay you.

For you who call yourself sporty
because you watch a game on Sunday.

For you who cheat at golf.
For you who run from tipping
because it might "offend" the waiter.

For you who stopped loving
because life hurt you too much.

For you who have no time to play with your child —
and end up sitting alone
because now they have no time for you.

For you skiing while others sleep.
For you sleeping while others ski.

For you who were off-key in music class —
and are still off-key in life.

For you who only hire people
willing to sell their souls.

For you who didn't give up your seat
for an old man on the tram —
because you just didn't see him.

For you who criticize Trump —
but God forbid Trump criticizes you.

For you who won't buy Viagra
because insurance won't cover it —
then wonder why your wife cheats.

For you who cheat on your wife —
because a buddy gave you Viagra
and now you don't know where to unload all that change.

For you who shop at the supermarket
to save a little —
then die sooner from all that toxic food.

Congrats. You really did save money.

For you who won't forgive your husband —
but still agree with Clinton.

For you who side with Starr —
but sleep with your sister-in-law.

For you who read every newspaper
to form an opinion.

For you who don't read a damn thing —
and still have one.

For you with no books in the house —
but a TV in every room.

For you who freaked out when the power went out.

For you who only started living
when the lights went dark.

For you who'd have been a Republican
if you were born in Long Island.

For you who'd have been a Democrat
if you were born in Greenwich.

For you who park in the disabled spot.

For you with the handicap sticker
but healthy as a fish.

For you truly handicapped —
but without connections to get a spot.

For you who give your church tax money —
then rape children —
because hey, Roman emperors did it too.

For you calling yourself "skeptical" —
because it sounds cooler than "ignorant."

For you who have cancer —
and won't die from it.

For you who didn't have cancer —
but practically invited it in.

For you waiting for scientific proof —
but at midnight, you'll still turn into a pumpkin.

For you who still believe in Prince Charming.

For you who *are* Prince Charming —
and forgot it.

For you, the postman who doesn't ring even once.

For you who complain the post office doesn't work.

For you growing an organic garden —
while smoking two packs a day.

For you who think eating rabbit
is more civilized than eating cat.

For you who roll your eyes
at someone on a diet —
but never had the guts to start one yourself.

For you who always want to be first —
and may only be blessed when you finally come last.

For you who listen to Jim Croce—
because he's dead.

For you who think Diana died by accident.
And that Kennedy was better than Clinton.

For you searching for America
while standing right in the middle of it.

For you Americans —
searching for America over here.

For *us* —
who stayed up till 2AM
just to write this lament.

The Imperil Syndrome

"A new day dawns upon the earth,
this hour is not a current, but a whirlwind.
Each personal world reflects the burning sky
for the fire that devours the old forms.
The wisdom of the Creator is a prophecy of a new world.
By destroying he creates"

Agni Yoga – Atarva veda

Theosophists coined an interesting neologism that fuses hate and envy into a single, corrosive force: *Imperil* — a term they considered even deadlier than AIDS. *Imperil* is the true evil of this century. And the only real antidote to this rampant plague? Forgiveness.

Forgiveness increases harmony. It seeps into you like light into dark water, rewiring your thinking and tuning your subconscious to the frequency of healing — to that cosmic love that permeates and binds all things.

Never forget this: the ancestor of every action is a thought. Every human act is first sparked by an idea — a simple, anticipatory abstraction — from which form condenses and hardens into matter.

Falling asleep with unresolved anger or conflict in your heart is dangerous business. Negative thoughts and emotions left to ferment overnight create subtle resonances — toxic echoes absorbed by your subconscious. And in that vulnerable twilight of sleep, they seep deep, contaminating your personal quantum energy field (CEQI) and quietly laying the groundwork for illness.

As a child, I studied in a Catholic school. I didn't understand most of the sacraments. They seemed boring, trivial even — long stretches of forced silence and stillness during ceremonies I was obliged to endure. The very AIr in those moments felt heavy, leaden, suffocating. My young restless spirit, wild as a colt, strained against the bit, desperate to break free and run. I lived for the moment the recess bell rang — that bright, liberating sound that summoned me back to life, to laughter, to friends.

I never would've imagined that, almost forty years later, I'd revisit those same spiritual dimensions — but through a completely different lens: the medical one.

After nearly two decades of study, I reached an unexpected conclusion: monotheistic religions — and Christianity in particular, the soil I was born from — contain extraordinarily sophisticated therapeutic tools. Tools no practitioner of causal medicine should ignore. Consider the undeniable healing power of prayer. Ritual fasting. The profound act of confession.

Christ himself — perhaps the greatest healer to ever walk this earth — descended from a lineage of therapists: the Essenes. And before stepping into the final, most grueling chapter of his life, he didn't sharpen weapons or gather soldiers. He fasted for forty days in the wilderness — wind and sand his only companions — purifying and fortifying body, mind, and spirit.

The great souls who came before us — the Prophets, the Saints, the Avatars — Christ, Buddha, and others — all worked for the same vast, intergalactic purpose: to teach the cosmic laws of love and respect.

They knew: every human being has the right to their own sacred garden, where the fragile, luminous flower of the soul blooms. And no God is greater than another — there is only *One*, who lives within us all, and whom every culture imagines in its own image and likeness.

Can you picture the creative leap of a Chinese peasant in the Middle Ages, or an African tribesman from a thousand years ago, dreaming up a God with white skin?

At the turn of the last century, the Theosophical movement in India was stirring up jealousies — especially among Christian missions — for its radical, liberating message: a brotherhood of souls beyond race, caste, or creed. A movement fiercely opposed to sectarian dogma, promoting instead fearless inquiry and reverence for truth.

Theosophists had a simple credo: *There is no religion higher than truth.* And truth requires integrity. Integrity requires self-respect. And self-respect? That begins with honoring the temple of your own body — a necessary first step toward inner awakening.

Any skilled psychic could see this expansion radiating outward — visible in the harmonious pulse of your CEQI, that vibrant matrix where true life flows. As Martial wrote in his immortal *Epigrams*: *"Living isn't surviving — it's thriving in full health."*

But many of us drift through life like debris in a river — fixated on dodging the next rock or whirlpool, oblivious to the roaring waterfall just ahead. Lives wasted in the frantic accumulation of the trivial, blind to the true riches of the soul. And when the final boarding call comes? You'll find that life allows only hand luggage.

Making a bold move before the current sweeps you away is terrifying at first. Things won't go smoothly right away. They never do. But success comes to those who hold on, who outlast the storms, who keep their eyes on distant horizons while others scramble for the shore.

As the Gospels remind us: *"God delays, but does not deny."* So why wait passively for fate to play its hand? Why not move now — confident, awake, and fully engaged in your own evolution?

I remember, during my teaching years in Australia at the Oceania College of International Nutrition in Brisbane, I met Henry Oziekj — one of the wealthiest men on the continent. He once told me that every serious life plan deserves *at least* five years of hard, strategic work — not idle waiting, not wishful thinking, but clear, disciplined action.

And what applies to one man applies to all of humanity.

So here's your call to action: evaluate your past, your present, your future. Take stock. Dream bigger. Plan wilder. And then move — unreservedly, unapologetically — toward the life waiting for you on the other side of fear.

Most of the diseases and afflictions that plague human life — obesity, diabetes, colitis, heart disease, dyslipidemia, depression, cancer — all spring from the same root: the inability to think long-term. We trade the future for the fleeting, chasing short-term goals like moths to a flame.

But it's the small, steady, conscious adjustments — the tiny rudder shifts — that allow a wise helmsman to navigate storms, harness the winds of fate, and keep the ship of life on course.

Look around. The endless crises USA have faced — from the Watergate scandal of 1972, to pensions, healthcare, education — all born from the same tragic flaw: the inability to plan for the long haul. Replaced instead by the greed of a few short-sighted rulers, ready to sacrifice the dreams and dignity of many for their own quick, conspicuous gains.

Selfishness is a disease. Not so different from cancer. It spreads best in dry, barren soil, stripped of oxygen and love.

But don't forget — each of you is a spiritual being, simply passing through physical experiences, moving from body to body with more ease than changing clothes.

Water that secret inner garden of yours. Protect it. Guard it from the constant assaults — subliminal and not — of media violence, consumerist noise, and the vulgar, blaring rage of a world disconnected from its soul. Every image, every headline, every ad hooks you directly to the darkest caverns of the human psyche.

Good and evil? Just two faces of the same eternal coin. Life itself is forged in their endless dance, expressed through the wild card of human free will.

Which spring are you drinking from?

One thing's for sure: negative emotions don't exactly nourish health or happiness.

Even on a purely physical level, professional "haters" pay a price. Their immune systems betray them. Their T-lymphocytes — the elite soldiers of the immune defense — lose their pseudopods (tiny feet-like structures that allow them to move freely through the bloodstream), becoming sluggish and ineffective.

Salivary IgA antibody levels also drop in these individuals — while those who choose forgiveness as a way of life display far stronger immune resilience.

Traditional Chinese Medicine has been saying this for centuries: feeding anger, resentment, hatred, and bitterness burns through the energy of the gallbladder meridian. The results? Migraines. Joint pain. Irritability. And a subconscious that starts writing disaster into your destiny.

Now — imagine the universe as an endless, boundless ocean. You can draw from it whatever you like. The ocean doesn't care if you come with a thimble or an oil tanker. It's always full.

But the size of your container? That's up to you.

Ask yourself honestly: *With what spirit are you filling your universe?*

Your subconscious self-worth determines the size of your cup. No one else.

Choose wisely, dear reader. Teaspoon or tanker?

Because the universe is never scarce.

It only waits.

Only Those Who Think They Can

"Those who repress desire,

they do it because their desire

it is weak enough to be repressed."

William Blake, - The Marriage of Heaven and Hell

Only those who believe they can — as Virgil wisely said — are capable of transcending. Through Panfhealing®, you'll uncover the power to shatter the limiting beliefs that have held you back from the success, wealth, and happiness that are your birthright. These gifts were granted to you the moment you came into this world, as a soul worthy of Love. Rediscovering your worth means forgiving, finding the keys to your lost paradise, and draping yourself in the glory you were always meant to wear.

Let those who've wronged you feel the warmth of your forgiveness. Release the past, letting it flow away like a river, so that for one fleeting moment, your hearts might touch — the moment of compassion, mercy, and grace. And when the time comes, bid them farewell, letting them go graciously to a brighter destiny. It will work. It always does.

Through this journey, you'll learn that true forgiveness cannot exist without self-forgiveness.

In fact, many lifetimes may not be enough to fully understand how to forgive yourself — but when you do, you unlock the gates of healing. Embrace life's lessons, even when they bring pain or suffering, and seek the silver lining in every experience. There is always a flower amidst the dung.

Allow yourself to surrender to suffering, for it is only through this surrender that transformation can begin. By facing your pain directly, you open the gateway to love. Keeping your heart open allows you to experience both joy and pain, knowing that amidst it all, there is an atoll of incomparable vulnerability and softness waiting for you. Seek it.

In truth, your vulnerability is your greatest strength.

Be gentler with yourself, and with life. Structural rigidity is never rewarded in this realm. When we resist, suffering only grows, becoming more vengeful and lasting far longer than it ever should. There's a saying in Alcoholics Anonymous: *you have to hit rock bottom before you're ready to seek help*. In Panfhealing®, you'll dive deep into your emotions, pulling them out from their hidden corners, and seeing them for what they truly are.

In those moments of despair, when the mind short-circuits and ordinary efforts fall short, you'll open to the help of the Divine Force. There's nothing new about this. Your guardian angel has always been at your side — their wings large enough for you to feel their presence, though you may not have noticed until now. And they whisper: *"I've been here all along, and I'll never leave you, from now until eternity."*

Judith Of The Angels

"In Serving One Another We Become Free"

Engraving on the Round Table - City of Camelot

Even if we can't hear her, we know she's always there, quietly gathering information and offering guidance for those who tremble in the dark. The Hierarchies rely on her much like Her Majesty's secret service once relied on the timeless figure of "James Bond" — a constant force, paving the way for you to awaken the sacred connection with your own Angel.

In the past, a weekend spent with the Angels and Giuditta (Dembech — b. 1947, d. 2023) was an event like no other. It was eagerly awaited by anyone seeking positive change, especially those among us who wore the "blockhead" crown — those too afraid to see what's right in front of them, desperately avoiding pain. For those souls, the residential seminar on Angels, hosted by Giuditta, was an unmissable opportunity!

A seminar on Angels? You might scoff, wondering what more there is to say. But don't underestimate what cannot be seen with the naked eye. That seminar could have illuminated your life in ways you never imagined, helping you rediscover your own Angel — the one you've always had since your birth. Although many of you may continue to ignore this presence, it remains unwavering, patiently waiting for you to acknowledge it, even amid the chaos of a mind that is always on high alert.

Ancient civilizations were guided by extraordinary helpers — the Angels. According to Theosophists, during the 4th Atlantean Race, the Deity walked among men, and the Divine Kings reigned in Atlantis, in the City with the Gates of Gold and Orichalcum. It was only when mankind strayed from the sacred path that the offended Deity withdrew, leaving humanity with only a fleeting glimpse of the divine, casting us into the Valley of Tears. Yet, the final word had not been spoken. Someone above decided to leave a rearguard behind to salvage what could still be saved.

Thus, a contingent of Soul Commandos — the Angels — was formed to guide humanity back to the Kingdom of Heaven. Their mission was to continue assisting us, combating materialism, and awakening us to the call of the lost Kingdom of Spirituality.

According to Giuditta, the activities of angels and humans intersect on three levels: physical, emotional, and mental, with a constant exchange of messages and information. Vast legions of tireless Angels work tirelessly toward the Grand Plan for Humanity's Evolution, communicating through colors, sounds, and vibrations that can be perceived by those who manage to silence the relentless noise of the mind. This is achieved through mutual, selfless service, transcendental meditation, prayer, and actions that serve the common good. The legendary city of Camelot, home to King Arthur's Round Table, bore an inscription on its marble, which encapsulates the essence of the relationship between Angels and Humanity: *"In serving one another we become free."*

The purpose of these beings of light is to enhance inner hearing through mantric sounds and melodies, allowing us to hear the invocations of mere mortals and pour out divine energies for healing and personal growth.

Humanity has long since forgotten the practice of praying to Angels to deliver our requests to the lost Divinity. But celestial messengers are incredibly swift and efficient, delivering their transparent messages when we finally decide to send them.

So, don't give up! Send your help letters — the angelic postal service is faster than anything you'll find in Italy, delivering your requests far more efficiently than FedEx, trust me. Sometimes, instead of stamps, you might want to use symbols. They cost less, require no saliva, and carry cosmic truths that can be read by your winged companions — and a select group of advanced human beings, as noted by Lorenzo Ostuni, one of the leading experts in this field.

Giuditta, like Virgil, endured overwhelming physical suffering throughout her life, yet she was always there, ready to guide you through the mythical Hades to reunite with your Angel. It's curious how those who dedicate themselves to the cosmic plan and the good of the celestial hierarchy often endure immense bodily pain, as if they, too, are shouldering a portion of humanity's collective suffering. We thank Giuditta for accepting this burden in her chalice, not just for herself, but for all of us, asking for nothing in return. That, dear friends, is the essence of true unconditional love — embrace it.

As Giuditta affirmed in her best-seller *Gli Angeli fra noi* (The Angels Among Us — Ariete Publishing), any human being — regardless of size or significance — can become an instrument for channeling, collaborating with, and spreading the angelic presence among their fellow beings. The key lies in maintaining essential qualities: purity, selflessness, and altruism.

Though it may take centuries to form stable, reliable channels between humanity and the Divine, the time is now ripe to begin. Now, it's your turn.

Giuditta remains, even now, a sister, a companion from ancient lives, and you'll feel a nostalgic longing when you think of her. How strange is the feeling when you first met her… a deep sadness for those who never had the chance to know her while she was alive.

"If you understand now, where is what you didn't understand before? What once eluded you is now being illuminated. And what now shines in your eyes is what once slipped through your grasp."
— Shu-chou

Transmutation Power Of Prayer And Meditation

You pray in anguish and in need;
I would like you to pray
even in the fullness of joy
and on days of plenty.
When you pray, you rise up
to meet in the AIr
the ones you can't meet
if not in prayer.
Therefore, your visit
invisible at that time
have no other purpose than ecstasy
and the sweet communion.
For if you enter the temple
just asking, you will not receive;
and if you enter to humble yourself,
you will not be lifted up;
and if you also enter
to ask for the good of others,
you will not be heard.

Suffice it simply
enter the invisible realm

The Prophet - Gibran Kahlil Gibran

Now, this might sound a little self-centered at first — as if prayer were merely a tool for personal gain. But the truth is, the human personality — the conscious Ego — is rarely in harmony with the Spirit-Self, or the True Self. More often than not, the little ego either ignores or outright denies the existence of this deeper Self.

Picture it like this: the tug-of-war between the personal ego and the True Self is like a person walking a stubborn dog. The dog (the personal ego) pulls wildly on the leash, determined to go its own way, while the owner (the Spirit-Self) pulls in the opposite direction, trying to bring it back on track.

This "dog" is wild, rebellious, deaf to advice, and resistant to the subtle inner nudges meant to guide it toward responsibility and wisdom. Anyone who tries to "pray" — or even take this metaphorical dog for a walk — without addressing this inner split is pretty much setting themselves up for frustration.

Only when the personal ego and the Spirit-Self learn to walk together, aligned and in conversation with a higher Divine source, does prayer become truly powerful. It's no longer driven by personal convenience, but by the will-to-good.

And perhaps, only when mystics, scientists, and philosophers realize they are all talking about the same reality — observing it from different angles but converging on the same Absolute — will the true power of prayer be fully understood.

Prayer is not optional. It's a birthright. And thank heavens, it's still untaxed — not even by Trump or anyone else like him.

Why does prayer work? Well, that secret might still lie tangled somewhere in the labyrinth of equations that quantum physics hasn't cracked yet. In the meantime, as the old saying goes: Don't look a gift horse in the mouth. Just use it. Let it work its magic, without overthinking it to death.

But there's a catch.

Prayer demands coherence. Integrity. Alignment. It's not a magic lamp that grants every wish — especially not wishes that disrupt the balance of the universe. So, if you're secretly hoping to cheat or profit at someone else's expense and it doesn't work out... maybe take that as a cosmic clue, rather than a failure of prayer.

Here's the thing: launching a prayer from the wrong platform is like trying to launch a rocket with the parking brake on. It's not going anywhere.

In this sense, according to Rose and Spindrift, prayer and meditation contain their own built-in regulating mechanism — a kind of antivirus — to prevent misuse and ensure they don't push an organism beyond what's truly good for it.

This "Guarantor" of prayer seems to take into account not only the needs of the individual, but also those of the community they belong to — according to an unwavering cosmic coherence.

But who decides what's truly needed — for you, or for the collective? A good Theosophist might tell you: that principle has always been at work, silently fulfilling humanity's real needs, whether we realize it or not.

When used coherently and synergistically — especially by healing or meditation groups — prayer can develop a laser-like focus capable of transcending distance and matter. It can generate a power for healing and transformation beyond anything you could bottle in a pill.

Meditation and prayer, when combined with creative visualization — practiced consistently and in harmony by motivated people — could offer an extraordinary working hypothesis for healing groups everywhere. Many don't yet realize that, beyond cells, membranes, and mitochondria, life moves along invisible wires, orchestrated by a Divine presence closer than we often dare to believe.

It's common practice in holistic healing to encourage those who are suffering to use specific prayer formulas — simple, sincere, but powerful — to speed up healing and deepen its effects.

For this reason, in the medical history forms I give my patients, I've included a special section with spiritual questions. These help me draw a more precise profile of their future self-healing potential — especially in cases of chronic or degenerative diseases, like cancer.

Here's a brief questionnaire you can include in patient medical records if you're a physician — or suggest to your GP if you're a patient. You're also welcome to fill it out and send it to A.I.M.O. (a.panfili@AImo.it), to help us better understand the phenomenon of spirituality and its role in healing.

Your answers will be treated with the utmost discretion and used only to compile statistics AImed at rAIsing global awareness of the universality of Heart Medicine. If you prefer to remain anonymous (in line with current privacy laws), feel free to leave out your personal data and use a nickname or pseudonym instead.

Throw your stone into the pond of intentions. Every gesture counts. Every effort adds up. That's how we change the world.

This form seems like a spiritual questionnaire designed to

understand someone's personal beliefs, practices, and experiences with spirituality and healing. Here is a revised version of the form for better clarity and flow:

Personal Information

- **Name:** ________________________________
- **Surname:**________________________________
- **Address:** ________________________________
- **Profession:** ______________________________

Spiritual Profile

- **Do you consider yourself a believer?**

  (Yes / No / Other)

  ____

- **Are you a practicing believer?**

  (Yes / No / Occasionally / In your own way)

  ____

- **Do you believe in the existence of a Guardian Angel or spiritual guide?**

  (Yes / No / Unsure)

  ____

- **Have you ever experienced contact with this presence?**

  If so, would you like to share how and when?

  ____

  ____

  ____

- **Do you practice meditation or prayer?**

  If yes, how often and for how long?

  (Daily / Twice daily / Occasionally / Only in certain moments)

  Please specify:

  ____

  ____

- **Do you participate in prayer or meditation groups?**

  (Yes / No / Occasionally)

  If yes, what kind?

  ____

- **Have you ever personally witnessed or experienced an extraordinary healing?**

  If yes, what happened?

  ____

  ____

- **Have you ever had an out-of-body experience, near-death experience, or awareness outside of physical perception?** For example, during an accident, surgery, or deep meditation. Would you like to share it?

This passage elegantly explores the interplay between spirituality and healing, emphasizing the power of faith and surrender in the process. Here's a refined version, maintaining the original message but tightening the flow:

On the Power of Spiritual Healing

One of the most astonishing observations we've made is this: Those who nurture an intense, sincere spiritual life—regardless of its form—seem to heal faster, with fewer remedies, and sometimes even without the need for conventional medicine.

Is it the power of suggestion? Perhaps. Or perhaps not. Who can say for certain? We don't claim to have all the answers; we're simply humble witnesses to these great mysteries.

But what we do know is this: healing happens. And sometimes, it unfolds in ways that science alone cannot explAIn.

"Thy will be done."

— Perhaps the most profound line ever whispered in prayer. It's not a surrender of weakness, but of wisdom.

So, write your intention. Cast it into the vast ocean of the Invisible. Trust the current. The vessel of healing will come.

What continues to amaze us is that those with a deep spiritual life tend to heal faster, often needing fewer remedies, and frequently without allopathic medicine at all.

Is it the power of suggestion, you might ask? Maybe yes, maybe no—who's to say for sure? Certainly not us humble, flawed mortals. But in the end? If the patient heals, that's what truly matters.

In the *Pater Noster* (the Lord's Prayer), perhaps the most complete and powerful prayer ever spoken by human lips, there's that crystalline, almost surgical phrase: *"Thy will be done."* Here, we surrender ourselves—trusting and opening ourselves up to that supreme regulating force.

The real task? Craft your request carefully, send it off with hope, like a castaway setting a message adrift in a bottle... and then wait for the rescue ship.

Because—trust me—it will come.

I asked God for strength, that I might achieve greatness;
I was made weak, that I might learn humility and obedience.
I asked for health, that I might do great things;
I was given illness, that I might learn to do better things.
I asked for riches, that I might be happy;
I was given poverty, that I might grow wise.
I asked for power, that I might earn the prAIse of men;
I was given weakness, that I might feel my need for God.
I asked for all things, that I might enjoy life;
I was given life, that I might enjoy all things.
I received nothing I asked for — but everything I had hoped for.
Almost despite myself, my unspoken prayers were answered.
I am, among all men, truly blessed.

Prayer of an unknown Confederate soldier. (The Oxford book of prayer - Oxford University Press, New York, 1985, p. 119)

Physiology Of Prayer And Mt

"A single thankful thought lifted up to heaven is the most perfect of prayers."

Lessing Minna of Barnhelm

To live in health—if we may borrow a line from Jovanotti, the iconic Italian singer-songwriter—you need a daily dose of positivity that springs from an alkaline body. Instead of throwing money into stocks and nervously watering your financial garden while waiting for a harvest, try investing in the wealth of the soul. Buy the only securities that don't fluctuate with runaway inflation: *Prayer* and *TM* (Transcendental Meditation).

You probably won't find them listed in the *Financial Times*, but that's hardly a limitation for the spiritual entrepreneur. More and more often, we see captains of industry, high-level executives, political leaders—men of worldly power—unexpectedly turning inward, searching for the roots of their interior lives. As if, at some point, the glittering narrative of wealth begins to crack, revealing the quiet whisper of a Faust lurking in the shadows, ready to bargain away the tired soul.

There's an ancient Zen koan about a young man on a quest to find the true Master, someone who could enlighten him about the eternal secret of life. As fate would have it, he meets a wise old monk just as the monk is pouring tea. Now, you should know—tea, in Eastern culture, isn't just a casual social or gastronomic event like it often is in the West. It's a sacred ritual. So much so that there's an entire ceremony devoted to this seemingly mundane act: the *Tea Ceremony*.

While the monk poured, the eager student launched into an impassioned speech about his life and accomplishments. But the monk kept pouring. The tea rose to the brim and then began to spill over.

"Stop! Can't you see what you're doing?" the student cried out.

Unfazed, the monk smiled, his deeply lined face full of serenity and light. "You can't fill a cup that's already full," he replied.

The moral is about as subtle as a billboard: when you're too full of yourself, you can't learn anything. To receive a new teaching, you have to first empty the container. That means letting go of old beliefs, suspending judgment, quieting the mental noise fueled by a delusional ego. Only then can you shift the lens through which you observe reality.

And how do you do that? Through meditation and prayer—simple but profound acts of inner power, accessible to anyone. They're the key to unlocking the greatest lesson of your life—the reason you're even here. The Japanese have a word for this: *Yoakhu*. It means "white space," the untouched background of an ink painting. In the language of TM, it's called the *Gap*—that sacred pause between two thoughts, the stillness between the object of thought and the thinker.

Many people remain unhealed because their domineering Ego drowns out the faint flame of the True Self, which lies coiled and hidden beneath layers of illusory identities. Pramandha once said that within every man lies a sleeping Master, waiting to be awakened. So let's start listening to that inner tenant instead of surrendering to the sly temptations of a culture that feeds us powdered milk and numbs us with painkillers, rocking our true awareness into a coma.

Too many have forgotten—or never even knew—that the key to healing is synonymous with inner growth. And more often than not, that path winds straight through the symbolic furnace of physical pain. Let's not glorify medieval self-flagellation à la Jacopone da Todi, but let's also not ignore the obvious: Mother Nature does *nothing* by accident. There's a reason she gave us over three million pain receptors and only about 280,000 for pleasure.

That doesn't mean life is meant to be all suffering, but it *does* suggest there's wisdom in pain—an evolutionary reason we're wired to feel it more acutely.

According to Spencer, it's not the strongest who survive, but the ones who adapt. And pain, if seen through the right lens, is a finely-tuned survival mechanism. It's a teacher—one that you don't want to muzzle with medication the moment it speaks. Of course, in critical situations, drugs save lives. That's not up for debate. If someone goes into shock, it would be *criminal* not to administer IV corticosteroids just because you prefer to brew hawthorn tea or reach for Bach flowers. In cases like that, science isn't the enemy—it's divine intervention.

Let the Buddhist principle of the *middle path* be the guiding light for enlightened physicians. The wise healer draws freely from all traditions—modern and ancient—without becoming a slave to any of them. The only sovereign is life itself.

We need to re-learn how to *listen* to what pain is telling us. Giving someone an antispasmodic for a stomachache could mask the symptoms of a burst appendix. Sure, you spared them some short-term discomfort—but possibly at the cost of their life. So, ask yourself: is pain really the enemy?

When a drug is prescribed solely to silence pain, it not only exposes the physician's insecurity, it also reflects a non-causal approach. And when you treat only the symptom, the outcome will almost always fall short of the hope for true well-being. Without addressing root causes, there is no real healing—just a superficial reshuffling of symptoms, like moving pieces on a chessboard. An illusion of change that leaves the deeper condition untouched.

Pain and illness have done more to unite Heaven and Earth than any philosophical treatise ever could. Without them, the two realms might never have spoken. Ramakrishna put it this way: "Illness is the rent the soul pays for inhabiting the body."

Fortunately, there's a growing number of doctors who are starting to listen. Some are even beginning to *prescribe* Transcendental Meditation—recognizing it as a statistically sound, low-cost tool for prevention and inner recalibration.

In the U.S., some insurance companies offer policy discounts to individuals who can demonstrate a regular practice of meditation or prayer. Why? Because those who engage in these habits consistently show significantly lower healthcare costs—fewer doctor visits, diagnostic tests, prescriptions, and hospitalizations. They also experience reduced rates of cardiovascular and degenerative diseases, including cancer.

Now, this doesn't mean that God has turned into a cosmic jukebox, dishing out blessings every time you drop in a prayer like a coin. Quite the opposite. Sometimes the jukebox doesn't play the track you selected, because true healing is orchestrated by an intelligent energetic field that knows exactly where, when, and how to act. It's like entrusting your life savings to a wise and enlightened financial advisor, saying, "Here's what I've got—do your thing. I trust you." That final moment in prayer—"Thy will be done"—isn't surrender to randomness. It's a leap into a cosmic intelligence that is both mysterious and just. Prayer works, but there's no cookie-cutter format for how it should be done.

In fact, a 1995 study at Dartmouth-Hitchcock Medical Center showed that among 232 patients undergoing cardiac surgery, those who found comfort in faith and meditation had the best survival rates. Non-believers? Their mortality rate was three times higher. Faith practitioners also had significantly lower blood pressure—by over 5 mm Hg—even when controlling for smoking and other risk factors.

Believers and TM practitioners also experience lower rates of depression, psychosomatic illness, drug and substance use, and suicide. In fact, among atheists, suicide rates are four times higher than among those who regularly attend religious services. Faith may support healthier habits—less alcohol, fewer drugs, more balanced diets—so their greater well-being could, in part, reflect a more disciplined lifestyle.

The mind is like a television with a thousand channels. To see clearly, you must turn the others off. "When our mind is focused on something, we become that thing. Contemplating a snowy mountain, we are the mountain. Watching a chaotic movie, we become that chaos. The channel we choose becomes the reality we embody—mind, body, and soul. If we light the flame of anger, we are anger. But if we ignite peace and joy—we become peace and joy."

When we focus our attention on a mantra-like sound, or a sacred image like a mandala, the body shifts into a deeply restorative state—the polar opposite of the fight-or-flight response triggered by the sympathetic nervous system. That stress response, while useful in an emergency, comes at a steep metabolic cost—it acidifies the body, drains energy, and accelerates aging.

But with TM and prayer, the physiology of well-being is activated. Heart rate slows. Breathing deepens. Muscles relax. Brainwaves shift. Stress hormones like adrenaline and cortisol drop. As a result, 75% of insomniacs regain healthy sleep rhythms, 35% of infertile women conceive, and 34% of chronic pain sufferers reduce or eliminate the need for painkillers.

In short: people who feel close to God, Buddha, Manitou, Allah—whatever name resonates—are not only healthier but heal faster.

We've all been carrying the weight of separation anxiety since we chose to incarnate in the womb. And so we reach out, through prayer, to reconnect. The biochemistry of prayer mirrors that of deep relaxation: it neutralizes stress hormones, lowers blood pressure, slows heartbeat and breathing, and initiates a profound internal shift.

This mystical experience unfolds in a very specific part of the brain. The amygdala—an almond-sized structure—works with the hippocampus and hypothalamus to form the limbic system. This region is deeply involved in emotion, spirituality, and sexuality, and through its intricate neural pathways, it stimulates the pineal gland's secretion of melatonin, which plays a key role in regulating the immune-neuro-psycho-endocrine system.

Neurophysiologist R. Joseph, at the Palo Alto VA Medical Center, has shown that stimulation of the amygdala and hippocampus can even trigger visions of angels or demons. In chronic drug users, these same pathways are overwhelmed—overstimulated by chemical shortcuts to states once only accessed through rigorous fasting, physical sacrifice, or spiritual devotion. Interestingly, both pharmacological and cancer patients report higher rates of religious or mystical fixation—evidence that suffering may naturally awaken these deeper faculties.

The pineal glands of long-term TM practitioners show superior vascularization and less degeneration with age. The ability to access mystical or spiritual experiences has a very real neurobiological basis, one directly linked to shifts in our body's pH. A more alkaline state seems to enhance our capacity for these peak experiences.

That's why monastic orders like the Cistercians ban animal protein—not out of dogma, but to prevent acidification of the body, which fuels the instinctive defense-attack modes of survival. Reducing animal proteins and refined foods builds an alkaline reserve—fuel for the very brain regions that allow for mystical connection and spiritual insight.

Modern testing methods, like ALITEST®, which screens for food intolerances, now make it possible to identify and eliminate acidifying foods that undermine both physical and inner balance. Of course, this isn't the only path—but it's one possible road. Healing is a process of awakening, of becoming aware. And yes, it can feel complex, even futile, to a traveler exhausted from the journey. But from the sky, to the aviator flying a thousand meters above, the path is perfectly clear.

It's a matter of perspective. The higher you rise, the further your gaze can stretch beyond the optical illusion of limitation.

This program is for those who are ready—who want to open their eyes and discover, right here and now, the paradise of harmony and balance that exists within. Every human being has the right to reach it. It's your penthouse. Whether you take the stairs or the elevator is up to you.

But when you arrive, you'll witness the most sublime landscape imaginable: your true Self.

Who Said Prayer Is Not Measurable?

"The truly religious man does not embrace any religion, and the man who embraces one has no religion."

Lorenzo Ostuni – Presentation of Biodrama

In his 1977 book *Methods for Identifying and Measuring Healing Energies* (Doubleday & Co.), Robert Miller describes a fascinating experiment involving an electromechanical transducer originally used at the U.S. Department of Agriculture by Kleuter and colleagues to measure the hourly growth of wild grass.

The device was surprisingly simple: a tiny lever was attached to the tip of a growing blade of grass. As the plant lengthened, the lever was lifted ever so slightly, and that motion was converted into a signal—recorded continuously on a slowly moving strip of paper, much like an EKG. The system was finely tuned, capable of detecting changes as small as a thousandth of a centimeter per hour.

Miller, intrigued by the possibility of remote energetic influence, reached out to the Worral family—well known for their prayer-based healing work—and asked if they'd be willing to "tune in" at their usual prayer hour, 9 p.m., and visualize the grass growing. Nothing fancy—just a bit of conscious intention projected from their home in Baltimore… over 600 miles away from Miller's lab in Atlanta, Georgia.

Before initiating the experiment, the device was run for several hours to ensure stable baseline readings. The growth rate was consistent: about 6.25 thousandths of an inch per hour. Miller sealed his lab to rule out any physical interference. Everything was ready.

At precisely 9:00 p.m., the Worral family began their prayer session. As if on cue, the grass began to surge upward.

The next morning, the paper strip told the story: the growth rate had spiked to 52 thousandths of an inch per hour—an 840% increase. Not only was this statistically dramatic, it was biologically astonishing. Even more interesting? While the peak subsided over time, the growth rate never returned to baseline. Something had shifted—permanently.

What had the Worrals done to trigger such an effect? When asked, they answered simply: *"We visualized the grass bathed in golden light and energy."*

At that point, Miller joked, "There's really no good reason left to be an atheist. You might as well start praying."

And perhaps he wasn't joking at all. Here at the edge of a new millennium, we find ourselves in the midst of a radical shift. The cold, mechanistic worldview of Newtonian science is giving way to a deeper, more integrative understanding—one that even mainstream physicists like Einstein, Tiller, and Lorentz leaned toward when they boldly proclaimed, *"God is energy."*

The ancient divide between science and mysticism? Crumbling. The Berlin Wall of the intellect has fallen. For centuries, the physicist and the mystic gazed at the same stars from different angles. Now, they're finally speaking the same language—and more than ever, they're ready to walk the path together.

As Baba SAI once said:

"The scientist studies the part of the tree above the ground, while the spiritual seeker studies the part below."

Both, it turns out, are essential if we want to understand the whole.

Rediscover Your Inner Divinity

The kingdom of God does not come visibly,

nor will it ever be possible to say: There it is or there it is,

for, verily, the Kingdom of God is within you.

Luke 17:20-21

According to Hindu mythology, there was a time when humanity so deeply abused its divine powers that the gods were left with no choice—they had to take the gift away. But where could they hide it, so that it would never be found?

From the heavens, the gods searched for the perfect hiding place. They considered the center of the Earth—but humans, relentless and curious, would dig until they unearthed it. The depths of the oceans? Still too accessible. Even the highest peak in the world would one day be conquered.

Exhausted by the dilemma, the divine council fell silent—until a wise one among them spoke:

"Let us hide the gift of divine power in the one place humans will never think to look: deep within their own hearts."

And so it was done. The gods sealed the treasure within us, and for millennia, humankind has scoured the lands, plumbed the seas, and reached toward the stars—searching everywhere but within.

Only now are we beginning to turn inward. Only now is humanity preparing to become an *intra*-naut—an explorer of inner space—ready to rediscover the sacred spark that has been waiting all along, quietly pulsing at the core of our being. But to do so, we must dissolve dogma, transcend conflict, and embrace the unity that underlies all races, cultures, and creeds.

This, of course, is not a new revelation. Over two thousand years ago, Plato, in his *Timaeus* (circa 410 BCE), offered a vision of cosmic harmony. He wrote that "the universe, or the great order of the world, was shaped by the Creator God as a manifestation and reflection of His own perfection."

We were always part of that perfection. We only forgot.

Now, perhaps, it's time to remember.

When Laziness Kills:

"The more you swallow it, the more...
it pulls you down!"

Guyton - Textbook of Physiology

The True Story of Joe and His Coffee

Taking medication to dull the pain of gastroduodenitis without changing your lifestyle is like turning off the red warning light on your car's dashboard when the engine's out of oil. Technically, the light's gone—but good luck keeping that engine alive.

That's why I'll never forget Joe.

Joe was an American engineer introduced to me by a patient of mine who worked at the U.S. Embassy. To protect his privacy, let's just stick with *Joe*. He left an impression on me not just for his nervous twitch or the fAInt scent of roasted beans that seemed to follow him like a perfume, but for his astonishing Guinness-worthy claim: Joe drank between 25 and 40 cups of coffee a day.

I did a quick mental calculation. If it takes at least three minutes to order, sip, and pay for a coffee, Joe was devoting two to three hours daily to his caffeine ritual. That's not a habit. That's a *career*.

At this point, coffee wasn't a beverage for Joe—it was his *profession*. Honestly, I thought my own mother, a fierce devotee of the dark nectar, was unbeatable... until I met Joe.

And yet, to my amazement, Joe wasn't vibrating through walls or trailing smoke like a steam engine from the 1900s. Even more shocking? He hadn't yet dropped dead from a heart attack or stroke. But life—and the human body—has its limits. Joe came to see me complaining of *severe epigastric pain*.

My first recommendation? Cut the coffee. Gently. Gradually. Not because I was worried about his palate, but because someone drinking *liters* of coffee daily can't just quit cold turkey without risking a full-blown withdrawal meltdown. Caffeine addiction at those levels is no joke—it's closer to coming off a hard drug than most people realize.

Clinically speaking, Joe needed a detox program and stress-reducing therapies—fortunately, all covered by his insurance. All he had to do was follow through. But when I explained this, Joe looked at me with a mixture of amusement and mild annoyance. He said he wasn't about to front the money—even though the insurance would reimburse him in a matter of weeks—because he was finishing the lease payments on his *brand-new Mercedes 600.*

And so, like a true caffeine warrior, Joe decided to keep drinking his 30-something coffees a day and just *mask the pain* with over-the-counter analgesics—the kind that eat your stomach lining for breakfast. He was convinced he was unbreakable. Immortal. I warned him: maybe his ego was, but his stomach wasn't. Nor was his bank account, once the real bills started rolling in.

Months passed. Then one day, I got the news.

Joe had continued down his path—coffee by the gallon, painkillers by the fistful—until one day his stomach gave up. Gastric perforation, peritonitis, and despite antibiotics and emergency care, it was too late. His heart—already battered by decades of caffeine abuse—couldn't handle the stress. A fatal heart attack finished the story in just a few hours.

Or did it?

Maybe Joe still drinks coffee—somewhere. Maybe in heaven or hell, where, if we believe the TV commercials, coffee's still part of the daily routine.

He left behind a wife, three kids, and an unfortunate legacy: not because he didn't know better, but because he couldn't be bothered to change. In the end, it wasn't the caffeine that killed him—it was the *mental laziness* that let it all continue.

No human being can guzzle a liter and a half of coffee a day without triggering very real, very justified physiological consequences—painful alarm bells the body rings to say: *"Stop. Something's wrong."*

Joe had plenty of warning. That pain in his gut? It was the body's version of the red warning light flashing on the dashboard. The sign that it was time to pull over, get a service check, and rebalance the overloaded system. But Joe ignored the light. He hit the gas.

And so, when his heart finally gave out, it wasn't some random failure. It was the body's last resort, its ultimate way of saying, *Enough.*

The truth is, the human body doesn't "get sick" in the way we usually think. It reacts. It compensates. It adapts—right up until it can't anymore. Illness is often not a malfunction, but a desperate correction to misuse.

No serious physiologist would ever claim that optimal human function requires industrial quantities of caffeine. Not a chance. Even the most advanced machines don't work that way—let alone the human body.

If you keep driving your car without oil and the engine seizes, whose fault is that? The car's? Or the driver who ignored every warning?

So, as always, we leave the final verdict to history. *Posterity gets the last word.*

Euthanasia And Therapeutic Result

"It is easy to descend into the Underworld,
but retrace your steps
and flee to the top,
this is the task,
this is the hard test!"

Publius Virgil Marone - Aeneid (the Sibyl talks with Aeneas)

When Joe (yes, *that* Joe from the previous chapter, for those just tuning in) finally came to me at the peak of his suffering, something in him recoiled. It's a common reaction. When someone like a doctor calmly points out that the problem can be resolved simply—say, by eliminating the root cause (in Joe's case, the coffee)—it often sparks fury instead of relief.

But really, what's the best way to stop your finger from swelling when you're hammering it on an anvil? Surely not by treating it between one blow and the next, but by pulling the damn finger away—or changing the direction of the hammer.

You might rightly ask: what strange, unspoken force drives a person to consult another flawed, finite human being (often even more confused than they are), and pay them handsomely for advice they likely won't follow?

Mysteries of the human psyche. Maybe the financial offering itself becomes part of the ritual, a placebo for recovery—*if*, that is, the money is more valuable than the habit you're trying to quit. Otherwise, even the sacred act of bank withdrawal loses its healing power.

So the question is: if Joe had loved his money more than his damned coffee, would he have saved himself? Maybe. Maybe not. Money can't buy everything, sure—but its loss can pierce even the coldest, most stubborn hearts.

When we suffer, logic and reason can backfire. We start to believe no one can truly help us. For some, it's etched in bold karmic letters that they must hit rock bottom to rediscover who they are—even if that completely upends the doctor's tidy ego, trained to fix what's broken in the physical world, not to wade into the soul's elusive, thin-Aired territory where medicine becomes a spiritual art.

It's like that story I once heard: An old woman, weary at a traffic light, gets swept up by an overeager Boy Scout desperate to fulfill his daily good deed. He grabs her by the arm, hauls her across the street with a proud sense of purpose, only for the poor woman—now stranded on the wrong side—to turn to a stranger and beg to be helped *back* across. Why? Because she'd been on her way to meet her best friend, who was waiting on the other side.

There's something telling in that image. In this metaphor, the "friend" is death. And maybe—just maybe—it's not always an enemy. Sometimes it's a natural, even liberating appointment, part of the great cosmic schedule. The body, drained of fuel, begins the process of letting go. And from a cellular point of view, death may be the most efficient exit strategy. It's the final surrender to entropy.

The point is: not every old lady crossing the street wants to be saved.

When I was fresh out of med school, the thought of saving a life lit me up with purpose. Even today, it does. But over the years, I've begun to ask myself—*really ask myself*—whether it's always right to intervene. If a body tortured by pain is whispering its goodbyes, should we fight to drag it back, or should we quietly bow and step aside?

Yes, it's noble—essential, even—to preserve a life that still longs to be lived. But saving it at any cost, against the quiet wishes of a soul ready to depart, plunges us into what some have rightly called "therapeutic obstinacy."

And that, my friend, requires the deepest wisdom—and the rarest kind of restraint.

All of this, without even considering that diseases show up to remind us of our mistakes—and *only* our mistakes. There's a strange comfort in hopelessness—it feeds the ego's desire to remain at the center of the stage. After all, being told, "There's nothing we can do," somehow feels more dignified than being looked in the eye by an orthomolecular doctor and hearing, *"Your suffering is the direct result of your own poor choices,"* as I had told poor Joe.

And yet—it's true. You can't help someone heal if they haven't decided, deep down, that they *want* to heal.

This bitter truth tormented me in my early years as a doctor, unleashing wave after wave of remorse. Over time, I've learned to tame that furious tiger, but I still flinch every time a patient walks in, dragged there by a well-meaning spouse, sibling, or friend. I've learned: if someone can't even muster the will to buy a tram ticket, they're not going to buy into the journey of healing.

Healing isn't mechanical. It's a fragile, complex alchemy of body, mind, and soul—a sacred dance that follows the ancient principle of *solve et coagula*. It's a cathartic process that can't be forced, outsourced, or imposed. True healing is born from awareness, and that awareness has to rise from within the sick person—not from anyone else, not even the most skilled or compassionate healer.

When patients begin to understand their emotions, to name them, to let them flow, everything changes. That's the purpose of a Panfhealing® session: not to control or suppress what they feel, but to *transform* it. Emotions, when acknowledged, melt away like snow under sunlight. But fight them, repress them, and they grow stronger—like an avalanche gaining mass and momentum as it thunders down the slope.

In truth, there are no "good" or "bad" emotions.
There are only *emotions*—raw data processed through our senses and layered inside us, like calcium building up in the filter of an old water heater.

If we learn to read the signs, we discover something profound:
The illness already contains the remedy.
The body's crisis holds the blueprint for its restoration.
But you have to be willing to *learn the lesson*—to let the illusion of the old self crack and fall apart, so that from the ashes, the true

self can rise.
Just like a Phoenix—born again from its own suffering.

Healing is always possible.
But it requires something radical: taking full responsibility for your life—and your health.

Stop clinging to the idea of being broken.
Stop pointing at your pain like it belongs to someone else: *my neck, my back, my heart's acting up, my ulcer, my cursed elbow, my toxic relationship...*

Stop saying *"my"* as if the pain defines you.
Start asking what it came to teach you.

The Mafias Of Pain

"While you taste all the pains of existence,
Tense your efforts towards the means of getting rid of it.
Give up regret, seeing causes sad and manifest,
illusions and actions"

Kelsang Gyatso seventh Dalay Lama

Ever noticed how in the National Health System, there's no reimbursement for staying healthy?

Health maintenance isn't part of the business model—only disease gets reimbursed.

If your bloodwork is clean, your X-rays show nothing, and your organs are humming along like a well-oiled machine, the system has nothing to offer you—except maybe a sympathetic shrug and the quiet judgment of having "wasted the doctor's time."

In fact, if the doctor doesn't find anything pathological during the examination, the patient may walk out feeling disappointed—disappointed that they're not sick enough.

That's how upside-down we've let this get. We've turned the absence of illness into a source of dissatisfaction. Compare that to the old world.

In Traditional Chinese Medicine, particularly in the imperial courts, acupuncturists were paid to keep the sovereign well.

The job description wasn't "fix the emperor when he breaks"—it was "make damn sure he never breaks in the first place."

The moment one of those sovereigns got sick? The royal acupuncturist was dismissed on the spot, shamed, and discredited across the land.

You were only useful if you prevented disease, not if you merely responded to it.

Can you imagine what would happen if we ran our modern system by those rules?

Imagine a world where a doctor's job is to keep your mitochondria humming, your gut bacteria thriving, your mind clear, your spirit at peace—and where failure to do so costs them their license, their income, their status.

It would flip everything. We'd stop worshipping the specialists who arrive in white coats once the ship is already sinking and start honoring the healers who keep us afloat in the first place.

We'd invest in prevention, not reaction. We'd treat health like a sacred asset—not a backup plan when the body finally crashes.

But no. In the modern medical theater, if you're not sick, you're not billable. And if you're not billable, you're invisible.

Picture(body meridiens)

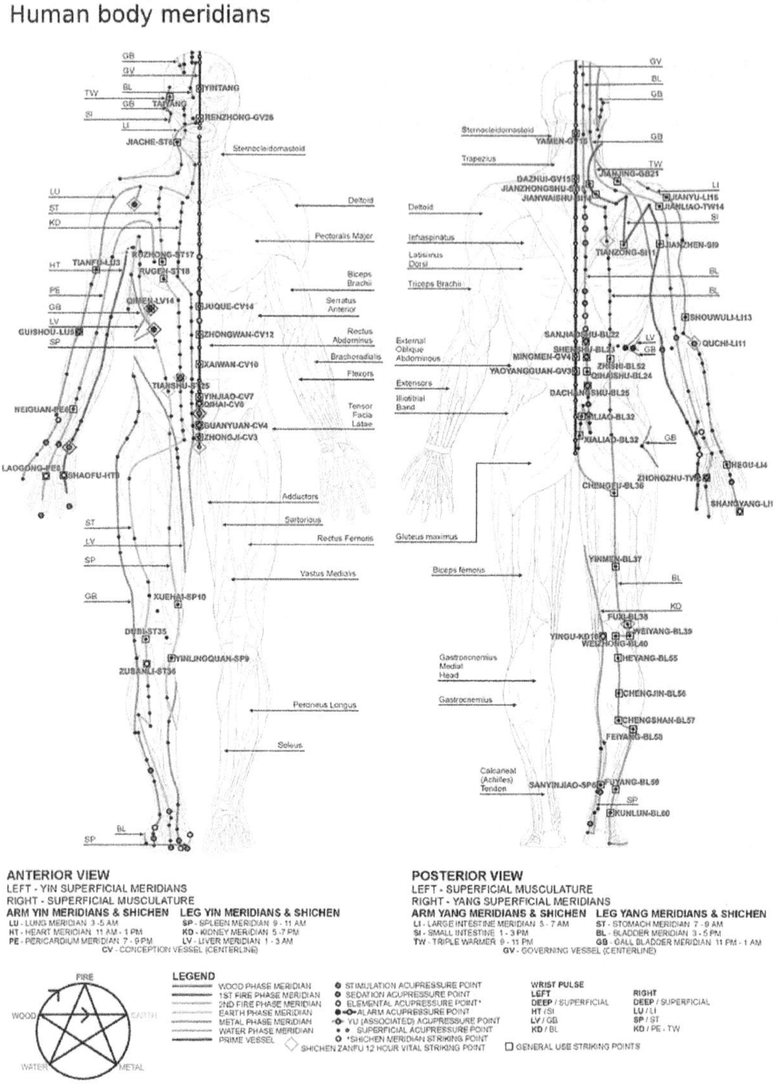

(Image from Wikipedia)

From Cold Hands To Warm Hearts: A Eulogy For Real Healing"

Healing, he tells us, is not a science, but the intuitive art of wooing Nature.

W. H. Auden

Who knows then who cured these Chinese sovereigns if they got rid of their healers so quickly at the first sign of a cold? Try to imagine what a wasteland it would be if this criterion of hiring and firing were taken as a model for public health. Let's hope the Health Minister never takes inspiration from the book you're reading…

It's not the doctors' fault that things aren't working as they should in healthcare, because the fees paid for a visit to a general practitioner, for example, are too low. Poor compensation for health professionals isn't beneficial for anyone, since, to meet their socio-economic and biological needs (even doctors eat, procreate, and go on vacation, according to recent studies), they are forced to speed up their performance.

Making a quick calculation, if a conscientious doctor devoted thirty to sixty minutes to a visit, he would hardly be able to pay for rent and other monthly expenses.

What should this hypothetical healthcare worker do? Perhaps starve while waiting for a politician to throw a few crumbs from the table of their endless banquet, reviewing rates that wouldn't even satisfy a novice in a Pony Express service?

In a fantasy medicine, which may not be as fantastic as it seems, it's clear that the weak link in the healthcare chain becomes the often-blamed general practitioner. In order to pay the mortgage and car bills that are due at the end of the month, they might be tempted to minimize the time dedicated to each patient, adopting mass-produced, impersonal medicine. In such a scenario, the anamnestic interview, thorough examination, advice, and the human empathy from which the final therapeutic solution arises might be placed in serious jeopardy.

In this context, it wouldn't be impossible for the humanity of the relationship to be replaced by blanket prescriptions for tests, medications, and surgeries, since the time available for diagnostic intuition would be drastically reduced!

It would also be illogical, should this unfortunate situation occur, to complain later if the health debt were to grow as quickly as a Christmas Panettone in the oven!

Many doctors are unemployed, and most are not only not rich but also receive, if they are lucky enough, a monthly salary lower than a very normal bank employee or public sector worker.

Furthermore, the freelance profession can financially support only a small elite of lucky individuals.

These considerations suggest that doctors are far more honorable than the tabloid press often portrays, as they never miss an opportunity to discredit a group of men and women who enter this profession driven by noble humanitarian principles. In fact, doctors often choose to accept a more modest income so as not to violate their Hippocratic Oath, which is based on mutual assistance and service.

Beneath each coat, human hearts beat, with all the strengths and weaknesses characteristic of this mammalian species. Therefore, it is unfair to generalize about the honesty of this group of Angels or Demons, focusing only on their mistakes.

Who knows why there's so little discussion in magazines and on television about those doctors who save lives through sacrifice, dedication, and passion, working tirelessly within the walls of a hospital ward, in an Emergency Department lost in a suburb, or at a field hospital…

Certainly, sad, upsetting, and painful news attracts more attention than the quiet work of love or kindness. Enjoying a negative emotion or unpleasant sensation is easier than it seems—just think that the most viewed films, those with the highest box office earnings, are horror films. The most popular television programs are the news, where pain and suffering are no longer fiction but a reality we inherit.

The information about the violence of a Mafia murder, a racial massacre, or a nearly lynched pedophile creeps onto your tables between a plate of spaghetti, a chicken jelly, salad, and coffee. It is digested and assimilated along with amino acids, vitamins, and minerals, entering your blood and reaching the deepest of your cells!

How many colleagues, in order to assist their patients, end up neglecting their families, their children, and contracting diseases between the beds of clinics and hospitals? How many of them die silently on the job, without anyone noticing or offering a word of comfort to ease the suffering of those left behind?

In memory of those brothers who sacrificed their lives for the lives of others, we ask you not to generalize and not to lump lilies and nettles together in the same bundle. Try changing your emotional approach with those who practice medicine, and you will realize that doctors, too, will change. You will enter into harmony with more real human beings who heal according to the rules of the heart and of love.

Abandon those useless and counterproductive euphemisms that almost make it seem as though those painful areas don't belong to you. Take them back into your heart, reappropriate them, even if they hurt. Joyfully, like the father of the Prodigal Son in the Gospel parable, when he finally returns home, even penniless and cold.

Regain your true inner power without relying on drugs, sharp scalpels, or expensive diagnostic investigations, because they are not always the coveted fairy-tale prince who can awaken you from the sleep of your despair.

Stop searching in Aladdin's magical lamp for the key to all your suffering. In this initial phase, a distorted sense of self often leads to transference (identification) with the therapist. If misused, this can leave the patient chained in ignorance and dependence, encouraging consumerism as a palliative of time, a substitute for love that was never granted before.

It's Not The Doctor's Fault

Much of humanity lives a life of gray and quiet desperation
disguising it with the pseudonym of resignation
while it is easier for a man to split an atom than to split a prejudice.

Occasional quote

Don't always blame the doctor if you are sick; instead, look in the mirror and ask yourself if you are truly ready to face the metamorphic experience of soul healing.

Some patients, just like many doctors, have their favorite diseases! Often, contemplating the possibility of recovery can disrupt the plans of those who live in mutualistic symbiosis with their pathology, as it provides hidden opportunities to gain affection and attention that would otherwise be unattainable.

Who knows, when you were little and stuck in those boring school hours that never seemed to end, how many times you played with a rubber band, rolling it around your finger? You must have noticed how the pressure from the coils was able to block blood circulation, making the finger pale, bloodless, and insensitive to pain. And when you removed the rubber band, the restoration of blood flow was accompanied by congestion in the finger and intense tingling and pain.

This principle is regularly applied in orthopaedic surgery to make the operating field bloodless (Esmarck's fascia). This mechanism closely resembles the behavioral strategy humans adopt toward suffering (remember poor Joe from a few chapters ago). When the human being suffers, it attempts to isolate the painful part from the rest of the body, forgetting it as a source of suffering, without ever bothering to loosen the tourniquet that has interrupted the vital flow, like sap flowing through a tree branch.

It would be enough to ask why a part of the body has decided to stop receiving nourishment, and with love, rediscover it to life, even if, at first—like when loosening the elastic—it may cause pain.

Pain is the consequence of your choices. Don't blame your therapist for developing unnecessary aggressive and self-destructive transference if you decide to submit to the "no pain" culture that the advertising media have falsely instilled in us.

Don't forget: the body is at the service of the soul, just as the car is at the service of the traveler. When the part you excluded finally comes back to life and starts to pulse, it may cause you pain, but since it's a symptom of vitality, you shouldn't be frightened.

Only what is alive can generate pain. When life stops, this healing symptom disappears.

So, the equation to rediscover is:

pain : waist = elastic : finger.

Patients involved in the intoxication of awakening their true self, resulting from the acquisition of awareness of the reasons for their suffering, often project their problems, emotions, and conjectures onto the therapist. In this phase, both the patient and the therapist must realize that it is not the doctor who heals in the patient's place, but the patient himself who rediscovers the thread of Ariadne that leads to his wholeness, ultimately reunifying the profound self, experiencing total well-being of body, mind, and soul.

The doctor is a minister of the divine that pervades everything, ultimately a humble instrument of what Hippocrates of Kos, the Father of Medicine, called: "Vis Medicatrix Naturae." It is important to recognize this together. Fragmentary phrases like: "Doctor, I'm much better, but my sciatica still hurts," or "I'm fine, but my diabetes still makes itself felt," reveal how the global self-perception of the being has been distorted and fragmented by the Newtonian mechanistic culture, which considers humans as the sum of isolated structural components (two lungs, a heart, two kidneys, a pancreas, etc.).

Redeem your true worth, for in reality, you are so much more than they've tried to make you believe! Claim your power and don't remove your hopes from the heart. Turn off the buzzing of your brain and rediscover the healing of the soul—the body will follow you docile, like a lamb to the stable.

In reality, the role of the therapist is much more marginal than patients might assume. Their presence and advice should act as a mirror of the soul, in which the patient can see their own erroneous areas, aberrant patterns, and destructive habits reflected—these are the unique and real causes of all diseases.

Only after a progressive and solid awareness, which passes through the expulsion of toxins accumulated over months or years, can the sense of self be regenerated and restructured to aspire to total healing. All diseases and all healings arise from the soul!

The body, the instrument of the soul, expresses a process that is often a source of pain and suffering, which cannot be hidden from the patient's eye. However, it must be confronted objectively, without frightening or demotivating the patient.

It is crucial to reiterate that the disappearance of symptoms to which one has become accustomed—due to the culture of medication—does not equate to healing. The pains that may arise when the healing energy bursts forth from the soul's source are precious allies, signaling life returning to nourish previously dead cells, tissues, and organs. However, the pain is not caused by the therapist, who prescribes a natural cure, but is the expression of one's existential karma, the consequence of one's mistakes.

Suffering is an inevitable cathartic element that may seem as frightening as the dark, bottomless abyss of the unknown. But, if you look closely, you will realize it is nothing more than a puddle a few centimetres deep. So, don't run away—look suffering in the face: the sad sister of the disinherited—and you will realize that from it, like the alchemy of the mill, the olive tree battered by the stone is transformed into living oil. Savour it, tolerate it, learn to appreciate it as a synonym of life. Having crossed the gallows of fear of pain, you will realize that it contains regular and constant rhythms that can be transcended and broken by recovering the total unity of the self.

If you manage to overcome this anguished crossroads, the doors of the Anthakarana (the gate of God, according to Sanskrit etymology) will open at the dawn of the new day of healing.

A key characteristic in these phases of intense prostration is realizing that pain doesn't hurt as much as feared. Anxiety and the emphasis on the expectation of pain are the true "idola specus" of Baconian memory, from which we must free ourselves.

Like the legendary Procrustes, the culture of non-pain, of do-it-yourself medicines for each symptom, has made you slaves to the ethical and intellectual tyranny exercised by those managing the so-called "pain mafias" (cancer, AIDS, chronic and degenerative diseases, etc.), who do not tolerate the judgments and actions of others unless they conform to their criteria.

"The more man weakens, the less he feels pain, while the most tempered spirits are also the least docile," Jack London wrote in his splendid book *The Star Rover*.

The spasmodic search for the magical genius of the lamp that can heal you is illusory and dispersive. It will be an endless wandering, Aimed at creating a distorted and evanescent sense of the true self, immersed and diluted in a surrogate of an elusive and fallacious transference with one's therapist. This genius often appears in the protean form of a white baron, or a religious or political leader, who, as the supreme panacea, can single-handedly unravel the Gordian knots of your existence. Even the pharmaceutical Robin Hood seems to be able to make up for this need. In fact, often, the sufferer places all his trust in the miracle drug, in the magic pill, thinking that it can erase days, months, or years of unconscious mistakes, like a magic wand.

In this phase, the seductive campaigns of the sirens of advertising certainly don't help, as they trap the modern-day Ulysses and his companions with empty promises of immortality. These advertising campaigns exploit psychological situations like these to fragment the true totality of each person. Antibiotics, like magic bullets, are placed in the barrel of weapons without safety devices, designed by a self-destructive society that puts the apparent profit of a few above the well-being of the community.

It is not excluded—indeed, it is very common—that a drug can get us out of a temporary emergency. The desire to take medicine is perhaps the most distinctive trait that sets humans apart from all other animals. However, it should be kept in mind that both poisons and medicines often consist of the same substance.

Finally, I believe that one of the primary tasks of the doctor is to instill trust and optimism in the patient, enabling them to regain enough self-motivation to assert and believe that true health can be achieved without drugs. For example, it is legitimate and desirable for a patient suffering from acute cardiocirculatory shock to be treated with cortisone, but once the acute situation has been resolved, the patient will need to ask themselves, if they want to survive this situation, the real reasons or series of wrong choices that led them to that conflict.

In this phase, Panfhealing® helps to take stock of your life, but remember that every synthesis brings something rotten and filthy to the surface, and this in 10-12% of patients coincides with the classic pseudo-aggravation syndrome.

Pseudoaggravation Syndrome: "Smiles Are Not Yet Taxable!"

Laughter is an effective and cheap drug, free of side effects.
While about 20 muscles are recruited for crying,
it takes more than 60 to laugh.

Adolfo Panfili – Daimon of Wellness, 1997

In the previous paragraph, we discussed how healing can sometimes coincide with a temporary aggravation of subjective symptoms. It's important to talk to the patient about this possibility, so they do not mistake this physiological situation for side effects caused by the therapeutic remedies.

How many times have we heard the phone ring, and how many times have we offered the same loving comfort to our patient brothers, assuring them that the body knows only one way to heal? We remind them to keep faith in themselves, despite the transient aggravation of symptoms that can sometimes arise early in the healing process.

The culture of medication has made people forget the importance of waiting for nature's physiological times to heal. Many demand immediate well-being as soon as a new therapy begins, and woe betide the therapist if the expected results aren't seen within a few days. It's not uncommon to witness patients, with arrogance and petulance, demand from their therapists an exact timeline for healing, even though, in reality, it's not the doctors who decide this but the patients themselves, with the help of the divine presence within everyone.

The disease process is slow, often taking months or years to develop, and it cannot be undone overnight with a simple solution. To heal, you must give yourself love—time and tranquility, which, like alkalizing tools, will carry out the rest of the work under your conscious guidance. This doesn't mean you shouldn't begin feeling better soon, but it does mean you need to listen to the true message of inner growth that the disease brings.

Time is one of the rarest forms of medicine in modern society, which has less and less of it available for the soul, and more and more for fleeting pleasures. Yet it is the great master, Time, who teaches the lessons hidden behind every illness.

Man can make a precise agreement with creative energy, deciding whether to use it for constructive or destructive purposes. Like a knife, this energy can be used to spread butter on bread and nourish you, or, when misdirected, can plunge its sharp blade into warm flesh, causing pain and suffering. Reality, like water, takes on the shape of the container into which it is poured. If God created the knife, He still gave you free will to decide how to use it. This, in fact, is the greatest gift He bestowed upon you: freedom.

Do not be confused if something inside you or someone around you suggests that God has left you alone. In that moment, He is leaning over you more than ever to help.

Avoid negative thoughts, for they crystallize the Individual Quantum Energy Field (CEQI), which must remain fluid and resonant with the rest of creation in perfect synergy and harmony to ensure health, happiness, and success. Thoughts are rarefied matter that can take on the coherence of a laser beam—so everyone must use them wisely!

If it were possible to fully see the destructive, acidifying effect of negative thoughts, we'd likely require a license to carry them around, as we would with a firearm. On the other hand, the thaumaturgic power of positive thinking—embodied by positive feelings, forgiveness, and love—is immense, which, as the Supreme Poet Dante once claimed, "moves the sun and the other stars."

However, as the philosopher Giambattista Vico would say, the history of healing repeats itself:

"When a man is ill and follows an unhealthy lifestyle, the first step is to advise him to change his ways. If he is willing to listen, further guidance will be offered. But if he is uncooperative, a true man and doctor would cease offering advice. To act otherwise would be to act like a coward and an ignoramus."

PLATO

As the wise Plato once claimed, he is remembered not for his thaumaturgical abilities, but for many other merits. And so, you don't need to be doctors, only logicians, to understand that changing one's lifestyle (hopefully for the better) is the first requirement for building a solid foundation for healing.

When washing a dirty piece of clothing, you've probably noticed how the water in the first rinse is cloudy, but then it becomes clear and crystalline in the subsequent washes. Healing follows the same principle.

When the body expels toxins, it behaves much like laundry being washed. At first, the water may look dark and full of impurities, which might make you grimace in horror as you consider the toxins you've accumulated throughout your life. But at the same time, you should rejoice, for you are finally expelling them.

When the human body can no longer expel toxins, it signals that the life force is running low. The excretory organs—kidneys, liver, lungs, skin, and so on—are so exhausted that they no longer maintain a satisfactory standard of living.

Pharmaceuticals, in this context, only serve to cloud the "washing water," acidifying the body. While sometimes a necessary evil, they offer a temporary respite, allowing you time to reconnect with life itself. In this time, the patient may rediscover the lost path to the alkalinity of well-being.

Love And Caresses To Lower Cholesterol

Accepting the evidence of the thaumaturgical capacity of touch,
of touching,
of the caress,
of sex,
of sweetness
it is uncomfortable and anchronistic thing e
scares everyone who
they barricaded themselves behind an electronic diagnostic tool
lest they love their patients
or who rely on the gelatin of a drug capsule
more meaning than a word of consolation for those who suffer.
What a nasty surprise for these lords of darkness
if humanity were to awaken from this nightmare successful and
just them should be at any moment ...
in layoffs!

Sweet and bitter reflection

Illness, in whatever form it manifests, is always a significant event—it marks the ideal starting point for experiencing love. Many healings are often delayed by a lack of love and time. The truest cure in the world has always been love; those who love deeply tend to live more fully and better.

To give love is to give attention, and therefore time. To heal, we need time—time that we often deny ourselves and our loved ones, and which the disease inevitably demands back with interest. Love and hope are far more alkalizing than an Alka-Seltzer. Offering them to others costs nothing and is immensely beneficial to both the therapist and the patient.

Even medical science finds itself puzzled by this essential aspect of health and love. Take, for instance, a singular scientific study from 1980 conducted at Ohio State University, published in the *Journal of Science*. The study involved administering diets with very high cholesterol content to a group of rabbits, measuring the resulting cholesterol levels and the degree of arteriosclerosis (hardening of the arteries).

What was sensational about the findings was that, strangely, one group of rabbits did not develop high cholesterol levels, despite being fed the same diet as the others. After months of conjectures and hypotheses, the discouraged scientists made an accidental discovery: the difference between the two groups of rabbits lay in the fact that the laboratory technician who fed the first group, a passionate animal lover, would not simply feed them; instead, he would take them out of their cages, caress them, cuddle them, and even kiss them before feeding them the same toxic food.

This discovery left the scientific team embarrassed, as instead of confronting the expected calcium and cholesterol plaques, they found themselves grappling with the unexpected evidence of the healing power of love. Touching someone with love triggers the release of specific well-being chemicals known as endorphins or natural opiates, which boost the individual's immune defenses.

Rather than acknowledging this, the team hastily labeled the incident with the misleading medical term "kinesthetic activation"—a curious neologism crafted to avoid the embarrassing revelation that a caress could be more effective than an antiplatelet agent or an antibiotic. But, of course, one could have simply asked any mother caressing her child: the power of touch and love is self-evident. Sadly, caresses cannot be packaged or patented by any pharmaceutical company, so it's better not to let that knowledge circulate!

All kinds of miracles are possible when one touches or brushes against someone with a specific intention.

Today, medicine has become far less manual and more cybernetic, with physical interaction increasingly being sidelined. We've forgotten what the great Master Jesus taught us: *"Homo homini medicus"* (man is a doctor to his fellow man). Our hands are the primary instruments for channeling divine energy, the true conduits of primary energy that doctors too often forget are part of their equipment intended to "touch" and heal their fellow man.

Nowadays, doctors' hands are almost exclusively used to interact with instruments and devices, and the essential physical contact—the caress, the so-called kinesthetic activation—has been lost. The fact that it was a laboratory technician who reminded researchers of the value of touch, something the medical profession risks forgetting, points to a deeper malaise within the system that warrants reflection.

Having sophisticated diagnostic and therapeutic tools at our disposal undoubtedly saves countless lives, and it's worth noting that medicine has made more progress in the last century than in the previous two thousand years. This explosive growth of technology, while invaluable, has caused some doctors to become over-reliant on methods like CT scans and MRIs—important tools, certainly, but not always necessary or appropriate. These technologies should not replace the simple wisdom of a well-placed urine test or a careful, conscious examination of a patient's symptoms.

Too often, the worth of a doctor is measured by the type and cost of tests they prescribe. But when it comes to healing, subtle emotional and psychological mechanisms are at play, and the economic aspect is not to be overlooked. However, it's crucial not to forget the importance of the so-called *"manu medica"*—the doctor's ability to perceive, record, and interpret the messages the patient's body continuously sends. Healing begins when the therapist becomes receptive to these signals.

Healing Hands of Light don't need electricity or batteries to function—intention alone is enough.

Yet, in the future, this might seem like a distant memory. In California, a new human rights bill could soon consider even simple acts like a pat on the back or prolonged handshakes as potential sexual harassment. What if, in the future, even smiles could be penalized for being too expansive?

Sometimes, a friendly glance, a gentle smile, or a delicate caress can heal more than any unnecessary drug. Listening to those in pain often soothes their suffering more effectively than an analgesic.

The most profound and magical moment is when a human being helps another—a spark of connection between the energies of two people, both working together toward optimal health. Humans are gifted with the divine touch of healing. When applied with intention, the act of simply touching a suffering part of the body becomes a solemn, powerful act of healing—an art form, blending the sciences of medicine and compassion. This makes the Daughter of Hippocrates unique among all professions.

In the future, when cybernetics dominate, perhaps we will call it the "medical keyboard"—a reflection of how technology has overtaken the simple tools of the human body. But what will the doctor of the future do when the power goes out?

They will likely rediscover the use of their hands.

Doctor You Saved Me!

More than by events, man is disturbed by his opinion on events.
Death is not terrible, but the terrible label we give it.
Problems, disturbances, anxieties are within us, in our thoughts.
It is foolish to blame others for it.
The wise man does not look outside for the cause of his misfortunes.
Whoever finds them in himself is half right.
Only he who accuses neither himself nor others is fully wise.

Epictetus - Teachings transcribed by Arrian between 117 and 120 AD.

In this phase of toxin expulsion, you may have begun shedding deeply ingrained behavioral patterns that, despite your best efforts, still feel like an intrinsic part of you, as if they belong to you like an internal organ.

You've started the journey of change, but you're like a child taking its first hesitant steps down a bumpy and uncertain road—the road to awareness. You may feel anxiety over the changes taking place and the detachment you're starting to experience. Much like a drug withdrawal, old habits will resurface in cycles. In these moments, you might seek help from your therapist, and they may seem like your savior. You might credit them for healing you, but in truth, the healing originates from your unique and exclusive potential. As Hippocrates wisely said, *the doctor cures, but nature heals*.

You may feel immense gratitude for your "saviour," whether it's the surgeon who performed your operation or the doctor who alleviated your pain. You might say things like, *"Doctor, I am grateful to you because you saved my life,"* or *"You have changed my life with this seminar,"* or even *"You are my teacher, and I owe my enlightenment to you."* These pleasantries are common during this phase.

But the true genius—the real master—is you. No one deserves the title of *master* more than yourself.

During this phase, the therapist receives honors and gratitude, which they may modestly refuse, recognizing that the true source of healing is life itself. The therapist is merely a witness to this process, not the giver of well-being.

Once you learn to silence the inner chatter of your mind, you'll find peace. You'll begin to sense the presence of the divine in your everyday life, both in the external world and within your own being. It doesn't matter what name you give to this divine presence—what matters is that you've realized it's there, and no one can take it from you anymore.

If you can catch a glimpse of this light in the twilight, it means you are on your way home. This is comforting, because while the journey is long and fraught with challenges, your true inner self will guide you.

Unfortunately, most of humanity remains trapped, endlessly circling back and forth like a hamster in a wheel, vacillating between two opposing behavioral patterns.

The key is to use your brain less and your heart more. Awakening through illness is a direct intuition of reality.

The Soul Care Session (Panfhealing®)

Hercules was assigned the thankless task of destroying the Hydra.
Each of his nine heads represented one of the problems that torment the brave who seek to redeem his soul through the mastery of one's illusory ego.
Three of these heads symbolize appetites related to sex, luxury and money.
The second three concern the passions of fear, hatred and the desire for power.
The last three represent the vices of the unenlightened mind: pride, separateness, and cruelty.

Alice A. Bailey - A Treatise on the Seven Rays Vol III: Esoteric Astrology Ed. - Nuova Era Rome, 1971

In Laos, after a serious illness, one is often allowed to change their name, perhaps precisely because the illness suggests a shift in perspective. It teaches not to confront the world head-on like an enraged bull, but rather to merge with the light of the illusion you are rediscovering by listening to what the soul, through its symptoms, wants to communicate to the oppressed and compressed self.

You are the one who determines the essence of your reality; you are the architects of your destiny. The cyclical nature of events — the perception that your wrong actions lead to stagnation in others' behavior towards you, and not merely to intangible bad luck — will gradually reveal the true aspect of the Law of Cause and Effect, which in Sanskrit is more succinctly identified as the Wheel of Karma.

Recognizing that the cyclical nature of the disorders marking your body is intimately linked to ancestral behavioral mistakes, perhaps learned through conflicting educational channels, will finally lead you to understand that it's time to release the guilt and suffering that no longer belong to you.

You are not overly responsible for the sins of your ancestors. Once you accept this, you will gain the energy necessary to change the world around you — if you truly desire it from the core of your being.

Think of the last time you were deeply happy and satisfied. Climb onto that cloud of joy, hold on to it, and read on, so you can return to walking barefoot through that secret garden where wishes come true if intentions are fervent… shhh. This is your silence, the silence of awareness, without which you can't even leave the house to buy the newspaper.

- Free yourself from the chains of suffering and symptomatic therapies that bind us to the yoke of disease.
- Consider every symptom and pathology as the true language of the soul, asking to be heard and freed from the labyrinth of psychotraumas that have built up in your being — day by day, month by month, or perhaps even years, stacking up in the dusty closet of personal experiences.
- New suffering accumulates, layering on top of the old, creating engrams in memory that influence the brain's sensorium, particularly the cortex. These engrams are ready to be crumbled by the fresh alkalizing energy of forgiveness, a true tool for complete healing.
- By spontaneously acquiring, within hours, a forgotten level of awareness and serenity through the synergistic use of ancient Vedic, Tibetan, and Taoist healing secrets, you will begin to feel the soul soaring light as a feather, after releasing old grudges and soothing ancient, acidic love wounds.

With these techniques, it will be possible to perfect neurophysiological functions by passing through seven main states of awareness. These states, according to Maharishi, are identifiable in ordinary states of:

1. CONSCIOUSNESS
2. VIGIL
3. SLEEP and DREAM
4. MINIMAL EXCITATION = PURE CONSCIOUSNESS or the GARDEN OF PURE INTENTIONS
5. COSMIC CONSCIOUSNESS

The fourth state, that of minimal excitation, corresponds to the level of Pure Consciousness or the Garden of Pure Intentions, where, if the request is pure and just, it is allowed to manifest. By regularly experiencing this state, the Nervous System adapts to a higher mode of operation, akin to shifting an already over-revved car into overdrive, allowing access to Cosmic Consciousness, where the state of pure consciousness is permanently aligned with the previous three.

Certain phases of nocturnal rest, meditation, and fervent, spontaneous prayer allow detachment from the physical body, turning it into a launching pad for expanding inner awareness through processes known as the "experience of the witness." This process allows access to goals that would otherwise seem unattainable. During these phases, the bioelectrical activity of the brain tunes into alpha and theta frequencies. At this stage, one can listen to the spirit that orchestrates the harmony of the universe, aware of the cosmic mind.

The progressive practical presence of Panfhealing® further refines this function, leading to the acquisition of two additional, even higher levels:

6. PERFECTED OR DIVINE COSMIC CONSCIOUSNESS, in which the spirit is perceived even within the object of perception itself.
7. UNITY CONSCIOUSNESS (fusion with the Illusion), where, as D. Epstein puts it, there is no one left to turn to, only the choice to dissolve into the depths of one's own nothingness — the final landing place, where God reveals Himself and intimate union with the divine is realized. This is the longed-for garden of inner silence where the psyche and mind are extinguished.

So let the waters be still and
You will find the moon and the stars
Within your being

— Rumi

According to Maharishi, in the gradual process of attaining higher states of consciousness, the state of pure consciousness begins to coexist and be maintained permanently alongside the other states of consciousness, even during sleep.

These states of consciousness have been studied through the recording of the electric potential fluctuations in the human brain, called electroencephalogram (EEG), invented in 1929 by H. Berger. However, it was not until 1957 that the technique was developed for this purpose by French researchers Das and Gastaut. They demonstrated that during a meditative yoga session, there was a clear increase in what are known as alpha waves. As the meditation deepened, these alpha waves were replaced by other types of brainwave patterns, including beta and gamma waves.

Particularly noteworthy are the studies conducted on expert Zen monks in 1966 by Akishige, Sugi, and Akutsu in Japan. These studies not only confirmed a unique physiological state on the EEG, characterized by a significant increase in the amplitude and regularity of alpha waves, especially in the frontal and central regions of the brain (a finding that was previously demonstrated by Kasumatsu and Hirai in 1966), but also revealed some fascinating physiological changes. During Transcendental Meditation (TM), they observed a marked decrease in oxygen consumption and respiratory rate, along with a slight increase in pulse rate and blood pH levels.

Furthermore, at the urinary and salivary levels, during the theta phases induced by meditative activity and fervent, spontaneous prayer, the researchers noted an increase in both salivary and urinary pH, indicating a clear tendency toward alkalosis (for more on this, see *pH Diet: How to Control Your pH for the Health of the Body, Mind, and Soul* by V. Mangani and A. Panfili, Ed. Tecniche Nuove).

Here is a revision with improved flow and clarity:

THE PHASES OF SLEEP

- **Beta Waves**
  14 cycles/sec – Wake activity with open eyes
  Typical of sleep onset, characterized by low voltage. Easy to awaken.
- **Alpha Waves**
  8-14 cycles/sec – Relaxation wakefulness with closed eyes
  These waves typically appear after the age of 12. They are necessary to receive psychic information.
- **Theta Waves**
  4-8 cycles/sec – Wakefulness in babies
  Very common in childhood and adolescence. These waves open channels of subtle interpersonal exchange and stimulate learning excitement.
- **Delta Waves**
  0.5-4 cycles/sec – Sleep
  Maximum restorative activity during sleep.

It is likely that in the phases of sleep, during Transcendental Meditation (TM), fervent and spontaneous prayer, or chemically induced soporous states (such as anesthesia for surgery or the use of certain neuropsychotropic substances), these specific wave patterns allow us to tap directly into the Akashic records. Through this, one can distill and decode firsthand information, which many artists, for example, have used to create art, sculptures, paintings, etc.

- Only those who forgive are in turn forgiven, up to the point where we realize there is nothing to forgive, because there is nothing to judge or blame.
- Realizing that we create everything we need in life: It is we, and no one else, who choose to create the hatred and resentment we feel toward others.
- Turning the other cheek should not be interpreted as an act of cowardice, but as a decision to view the future through different eyes, from the perspective of forgiveness. Often, those who suffer the most are the ones who cling to old patterns and mental attitudes, because change frightens them.
- Having someone to hate often helps one survive, but it certainly doesn't help one live life to the fullest. Rather than holding onto grudges for an injustice that can literally consume us, it is essential to find the positive side, even in the bleakest experiences. Forgiveness does not mean sharing the harm done to us, but simply letting it go out of self-compassion.
- Forgiveness alkalizes the individual, relaxing them and generating the vibrational energy field essential for this great and simple miracle to repeat itself. By giving others space, we also gain more Air for ourselves. In this regard, W. Goethe once said that to live better with others—a task that has always been

delicate and demanding, especially for those who struggle with their own self—one should: *"Treat others for who they are, not for what we would like to think of them."*

The Appointment With The True Self

"When you will be aware
of the fact that you yourself are a
miracle, you will also start
to be sure that
nothing is impossible for you".

Wayne W. Dyer – Everyday wisdom

Finding the words never spoken by loved ones who are no longer with us, allowing their souls to return to the ocean of energy from which we all come and to which we all long to return.

- Becoming aware that we are all walking the same path, seeking the true home of the soul.
- Discovering that truth is the key to healing, a key that is within everyone's reach, even if not everyone is able to grasp it due to mental laziness and reluctance to make themselves available.
- Learning to breathe in the awareness of the serene alkalinity of well-being, navigating the jungle of daily stress through an exclusive, full-immersion seminar on you, with a limited number of participants.

- No final diploma is conferred, for no one is a master except of oneself. The disease or painful symptom is simply the cry for love from cells, tissues, and organs, which are waiting to be heard. The best certificate that can be given is awareness itself.
- Pause for a moment to receive the **message** that every atom of your body is trying to deliver, and in the harmony of a collective group, learn how to find the true path of healing through Panfhealing®.
- Living experiences of inner regeneration, learning to uncondition the mind, which distorts and amplifies old conflicts stored in the brain's "hard disk," blending them with new ones.
- Finally tending to ancient, unhealed love wounds, which, like a grain of sand, roll down the slope of memory, combining with new psychotraumas to become an unstoppable avalanche capable of overwhelming everything in its path.

This and more will happen when you learn that the real miracles are those that you yourself can perform, rediscovering the divine spark that has always been within you, and through the chain of rebirths, you are learning to reconnect with it. By participating in the banquet with your true self, you reunite with the illusion that kept you separated from your light or your shadow.

- A final review of your emotional profiles and commentary on the orthomolecular precepts of Prof. Panfili will help you stay on course, maintaining the momentum, flexibility, consciousness, and energy that had been alienated, traumatized, or misdirected.

- Rediscover the awareness of your own forms and real possibilities, reconnecting with the external rhythms from which you were estranged, and transcending all the limits that were imposed upon you, which do not belong to you.
- Break through your limits and find your true self, here and now!

Disease Separates What God Has United: The Unifying Orthomolecular Function Of Panfhealing® @

"Before the soul can stand before the Masters, her feet are to be washed in the blood of the heart."

Alice A. Bailey - The Light on the Path - Nuova Era Editions 1971

The Panfhealing® session typically begins at 9 a.m. and lasts until 3 p.m., with two intervals—one mid-morning and another at lunchtime. During these breaks, an orthomolecular menu is recommended, consisting of 80% vegetables and fruits, with the remaining portion made up of cereals, proteins, and fats.

The Panfhealing® class incorporates movements, sounds, breathing techniques, Kune, yoga, MT, Best, Network, aromatherapy, Bach flower therapy, meditation, and crystal therapy. Each of these methods, when properly integrated, helps awaken physical and psychic sensations or memories. The process of healing during these sessions may evoke ecstatic or wonderful experiences, or sometimes, it might bring up feelings of discomfort. However, this is all part of the entrancing journey you are about to embark on. So, remember to bring a woolen sweater, as the coldness of forgiven memories might brush against your skin.

Healing is not simply about removing symptoms—it goes much deeper. True healing comes from the reorganization of how we relate to others and, most importantly, to ourselves. Illness separates what God has united, while healing works to bring back together and reintegrate those areas, tissues, and organs that have been forgotten. It's possible that this process can trigger symptoms or even pain—but that's all part of the journey, dear readers!

Panfhealing® provides the space and time we need to rediscover ourselves and better understand the messages that our symptoms are trying to convey. With this technique, each individual will seek and find the secret combination to unlock their own inner casket, where the magical formula necessary to begin restructuring their existence is kept.

It's possible that it's our repeated attempts to control the flow of experiences that create congestion of energy in various parts of the body. Surrendering to your deepest inner self allows you to reacquire, without inhibition, the natural rhythms of the soul, which will retune the out-of-sync strings of life's harp, like a magical tuning fork.

Rediscover this innate wisdom within, breathe it in deeply—as if after an eternal apnea. By embracing and transcending the symptoms, and through healing, you will rediscover forgotten drives and strategies, leading to a sense of self-satisfaction and strengthening unity within.

Approximately 20 people are accepted for each Panfhealing® class, where participants are encouraged to lie on beds throughout the session.

How To Survive The 3rd Millennium

"Before the voice can speak before God it must have lost the power to wound"

Alice A. Bailey – The light on the path, Nuova Era Editions 1971

Consider this text as a quick survival manual for the now incandescent third millennium. It's a simple, unpretentious guide, written by someone like you, who travels a road filled with challenges but also with fascination and wonder. It's a path toward meditative resonance with true inner healing energies.

These hidden and often forgotten energies are always ready to flow back swiftly and majestically through the body's meridians, at the mere nod of your understanding. Within these pages, you will find fundamental explanations of the various orthomolecular diagnostic methods used in Panfhealing® practice, including Alitest®, Canditest, TASC (testing for antigens against candida), and TMTU (testing for heavy metals in urine). These methods are instrumental in rediscovering the alchemical gold of total well-being that we all seek together.

I am not a keeper of ancient wisdom but a humble fellow traveler, much like you, trying to find the Ariadne's thread that will guide us back home. Together, we will seek to gain awareness in the health jungle, starting from the dental sector (such as dental amalgam poisoning), addressing controversial topics like excessive vaccination practices and their side effects, and moving on to the subtle physiology of healing energy, the therapeutic power of forgiveness, and more—everything that will unfold throughout this work of love and sharing.

Panfhealing® is the spontaneous awakening of the Vis Curandi, the healing power that resides in everyone's heart, waiting to be ignited—just like the tale of Sleeping Beauty in the woods. It is no coincidence that we meet again now… after all, coincidences do not exist, except for those too afraid to realize that the entire universe shares the same anima mundi, as Giordano Bruno once claimed.

The journey of the soul through the tangible worlds of the bodies it inhabits on its long pilgrimage from star to star does not follow a linear or continuous path, nor can it be constrained by rigid mathematical equations. Critical phases can interrupt this evolution, marked by real, qualitative-energetic leaps. These phases manifest with the shedding of the past, similar to a rocket discarding stages to reach much higher spiritual peaks. In such moments, death and rebirth coexist, much like the chrysalis before the butterfly emerges in its catharsis.

We AIm to create a unique opportunity with you—one where we foster harmony between awareness and healing. Most seminars often begin with a critical purpose but lack the practical tools to truly guide people toward inner transformation. This results in what is often called post-seminar depressive syndrome, where participants ask themselves the age-old question: "The teachings were wonderful, but where do we start now?"

Let's begin from Panfhealing®, here and now, all together, with a shared goal: to reconnect with our deepest selves, which will guide us through the process of inner metamorphosis.

The secret formula of Panfhealing® is that it's a concentrated version of this orthomolecular philosophy, expanded by the wisdom of Tibetan, Ayurvedic, and initiatory medical techniques. This powerful approach has helped many people heal quickly without the use of drugs, allowing them to harness their own strength and gain ever-deepening awareness of their chosen path. Treating numerous patients with this global system has shown significant success, greatly increasing recovery rates.

This success is likely due to what we call the "sanctuary effect" (a term coined by me), which occurs when a group of individuals, strategically motivated by positive expectations, is guided into healing sessions, often resulting in what outsiders might describe as "miraculous" recoveries. In reality, these are not miracles but rather the result of a mechanism known in electronics as parallel connection (the same principle used when bridging batteries to start a car).

The Panfhealing® session is focused on helping others directly, without unnecessary embellishments or idle chatter, offering precise and immediate solutions. It involves a series of modular adjustments across different sequential energy spheres, allowing the patient to experience firsthand, even as a beginner, the transformative peaks of TM experiences or ecstatic states in a very short time.

This process takes place in an environment enhanced by carefully chosen music and special transcommunication quartzes that, like dedicated Carthusians, tirelessly assist in the healing endeavor. Special emphasis is placed on mastering an appropriate and effective breathing dynamic, which is crucial for the process.

At the end of the session, an audiocassette is typically provided, summarizing the experience so you can replicate it at home. The cassette contains the foundational theory of the session and a summary of the book on Panfhealing®.

Panfhealing® Physiology

"Every student of nature should follow this rule: consider with suspicion anything mentioned the mind takes possession with satisfaction."

Francis Bacon

The physiological effects of Panfhealing® can be summarized, at least in part, by those induced through Transcendental Meditation (TM).

Gaining autonomy and reaping the benefits of TM is not a quick process. In fact, it requires a great deal of dedication, as the practice must be meticulously guided by an initiator until the student can begin to take their first independent steps into this relatively unexplored realm for Western populations. Though it may seem distant, it is, in truth, incredibly close—right at the heart of the soul.

Panfhealing® works much faster and is less tedious than the early stages of TM. It engages spheres of awareness, participation, and information that are more suited to the Western mind. Westerners often require a rational entry point before venturing into the deeper, hidden realms of inner exploration.

From the very first session, one can experience these profound inner peaks—initially thought to be inaccessible to beginners—yet they are already available to those motivated by the desire for healing, as they call forth love and well-being from their true self.

When disease serves as a purifier of egoic habits, it becomes, as Brother Francis might say, a blessing. It is a form of catharsis, readying the individual for this new season of life. While Westerners are statistically more prone to illness than their Eastern counterparts, we like to believe that they are also granted more powerful mechanisms for healing—like Panfhealing® @.

Think of it as the alchemical crucible of the 3rd millennium, boiling away the dross of disease to reveal the gold of healing. If disease had not been invented, there would be no health. Since health is a mental state, mirroring the temperature of the soul, there's no better way to restore it than when the noise of the mind quiets down during restful sleep.

Metabolic Effects of Panfhealing®:

1. 15% Reduction in Basal Metabolism
2. Reduction in Plasma Concentration of Stress Hormones (Catecholamines, Cortisol)
3. Reduction in Heart and Respiratory Rate
4. Reduction in Lactic Acid Formation in Muscular Tissue
5. Systemic Alkalinization of Physiological Fluids (Blood, Saliva, Urine)
6. The detection of additional significant parameters suggests a state of deep and widespread relaxation, including:
    1. Lowering of Hypertonus in Gamma-Motoneurons (responsible for muscle tone or residual muscle contraction)
    2. Improved Perfusion of the CNS (Central Nervous System) as evidenced by MRI (Epstein D. 1996)
    3. Increase in Electrocute Resistivity Measured by Functional Organometry (Voll method)
    4. Increase and Prevalence of Alpha Waves In the EEG trace

West Of The Soul

"God is forced to pour himself completely into every man that he has totally detached himself from the self"

Meister Eckart

TRANSCENDENCE, AND THE COSMOZOA THEORY

In contrast to Immanence, Transcendence signifies, in an active sense, the movement of surpassing or going beyond something regarded as a point of reference. According to the neo-Platonists, the One is considered transcendent even in relation to Being itself, and this view is echoed in various negative theologies which attribute transcendence to God.

Life on Earth emerged from physical elements with a carbon-based structure, defined as amino acids—the foundational building blocks of proteins (see *Orthomolecular Medicine: A Therapy on a Human Scale* - Ed. Tecniche Nuove). Your existence depends on these fundamental components, which form the very roots of human beings. These biological processes were inherited from your animal ancestors, who in turn evolved from the plant world, which itself originated from the mineral realm. These three forms of evolution—

inorganic, biological, and psychosocial—while sharing numerous common elements, operate according to distinct and transcendent principles.

Organic chemistry, for example, cannot fully explain the vital processes of cells, even though each of these processes is a result of chemical interactions. Likewise, zoology, despite examining the many parallels between Homo Erectus and the great anthropoid apes, is unable to account for the finer details of what makes humans unique.

In 1898, Arrhenius, in his work *Cosmic Influences on Physiological Phenomena*, proposed that the moon influences physiological processes such as births, deaths, epileptic seizures, and menstrual cycles in women. Newton's concept of gravitational interaction between the moon and the sun causes periodic, regular, and consistent oscillations in the seas, known as tides. These oscillations result in two high tides and two low tides during each lunar day, which lasts 24 hours and 50 minutes. This tidal rhythm is characterized by a period of 12 hours and 25 minutes, or 44.676 seconds.

Due to thermal convection in large Air masses, tidal dynamics lead to significant variations in atmospheric pressure. Remarkably, the rhythm of the human respiratory rate appears to resonate harmoniously with the tidal wave. This is evident in the fact that the period of human breath is roughly 13,000 times shorter than that of the tides:

$$\frac{44{,}676}{13{,}000} = 3.43 \text{ seconds}$$

Similarly, the movement of blood fluids in the human body seems to be in sync with the tidal rhythm. Following the displacement of massive water masses, tidal currents develop in the seas at a speed of about 0.5 m/sec, which corresponds to the flow rate of blood in the body: 10 cm/sec in veins and 20-40 cm/sec in arteries.

These observations suggest that both heart rate and respiration are periodic phenomena that are proportional to the speed of the tidal wave's advancement.

The Woman, The Water And The Moon

Being biologically richer in water than men, the female organism is more sensitive to variations in gravitational attraction during the lunar synodic month, much like the oceans respond to tidal changes. This sensitivity gives rise to the cyclical trend of the menstrual flow. It is no coincidence that the human menstrual cycle lasts roughly the same duration as the lunar cycle, approximately 29 and a half days.

Furthermore, the duration of pregnancy corresponds to nine lunar months, or about 265.8 days, as confirmed by a study conducted by Menaker in 1959, based on a sample of 250,000 births. Even reproduction itself appears to be marked by external astronomical rhythms, beyond the intrinsic biology of the human cell.

The position of the Moon in relation to the Sun is also responsible for environmental and behavioral shifts that have been recognized for centuries. Irregularities in these cycles are often linked to exposure to light at night, disrupting the synchronization of the circadian melatonin secretion rhythm with the full moon phase. In some cases, women suffering from dysmenorrhea can regulate their menstrual flow simply by turning on low-intensity lights during the night of days 14-16 of their cycle, avoiding the need for medication.

These are not just coincidences. They point to the observation that the physiological functions of the human body resonate with the Earth's vital and pulsating activity—an Earth that itself is a living organism, with energy that flows along preferential lines, analogous to the acupuncture meridians in the human body.

In his theory of cosmozoans (Panspermia), Arrhenius proposed that life could travel between planets through living microorganisms that could endure the extreme temperatures of celestial bodies. These resilient life forms would journey from star to star, fostering the transmission of life across the cosmos.

Extraterrestrial Life: We Are Not Alone In The Universe!

At the University of Illinois, astronomer Lewis Snyder reportedly discovered the presence of the amino acid glycine in our galaxy, located just one light-year from Earth in the Milky Way's Sagittarius B2 nebula. Glycine, also known as aminoacetic acid, is the fundamental molecule from which all 20 (or 22, according to some sources) essential and non-essential amino acids derive—the building blocks of life. These amino acids are constructed from four inseparable elements: carbon, oxygen, hydrogen, and nitrogen. Since both the human body and the nucleus of comets are composed of these elements in nearly identical proportions, it is reasonable to suggest that life on any planet, in any galaxy, must have evolved from this identical biochemical foundation.

In this way, hypothetical extraterrestrial life forms might share organic functions quite similar to those of Earth's inhabitants, whether it's Zac Efron or Paris Hilton, assuming chemistry remains universal. Imagine, for a moment, if 65 million years ago, the dinosaurs hadn't become extinct due to a catastrophic asteroid impact or a rogue comet. In such a scenario, humans might have evolved from dinosaurs instead of primates, following the theories of Lamarck and Darwin. It's not so difficult to imagine spending a weekend in Miami with a Tyrannosaurus Rex instead of the usual family gatherings... though it's hard to say if it would be a better alternative.

In the past thirty years, thanks to Radio Astronomy Spectroscopy (which analyzes chemical elements in the universe based on their electromagnetic emissions), the discovery of glycine has provided strong evidence for the possibility of extraterrestrial life. This confirms that prebiotic phenomena—the processes that set the stage for life—are likely not unique to Earth but are occurring throughout our galaxy. It might be unsettling to consider the possible simultaneous existence of several versions of celebrities like Beyoncé, Tom Cruise, or even historical figures like Adolf Hitler. But let's leave such speculations to science fiction, turn off the TV, and engage our third eye, for intuition often reaches farther than Cartesian logic.

Among the countless radiations emitted by who knows how many molecules, the specific wavelength of glycine was captured, marking the first fragment of the life mosaic. Hundreds of other spectral lines, like Pirandellian "characters in search of an author," await their chemical identities to determine whether they belong to amino acids or other molecules. Just like wandering travelers between stars, life, born in the alchemical gestation within a passing comet or inside a hurried meteorite, has come into existence—and will continue to do so.

Swarming comets, blazing across celestial paths, deposited the water that now forms Earth's oceans, along with carbon skeleton compounds essential for triggering prebiotic processes that would lead to life. Significant insights came from the 2003 Rosetta mission, which unveiled remarkable findings, including ancient icy water vastly different from Earth's, and the discovery of pungent chemicals such as hydrogen sulfide, ammonia, and formaldehyde emanating from the comet's porous structure. These discoveries provided valuable clues about the early days of the solar system.

From this, we can conclude that where amino acids like glycine are found, life may have arrived from distant corners of the universe and is still ongoing, has already existed, or will exist, provided the right conditions (pressure, temperature, magnetic field) are met. In the blink of an eye—roughly 300 million years—what was once inert matter transformed into vibrant life.

This brings us to the fascinating episode of the Apollo project, during which clandestine colonies of streptococcal spores were discovered in a television camera that had been to the Moon. Upon return, these spores were found to be in excellent condition, despite enduring the harshest conditions: extreme cold, cosmic radiation, and the absolute vacuum of space. While many scientists attempt to explain life's processes in strictly physical and chemical terms—rationalizing human awareness as merely biological—it will take more time before researchers across disciplines come together at the same table to truly assist humanity in understanding the full scope of life's mysteries.

SIRVAPP (Hypometabolic State of Parasympathetic Predominantly Supervisory Response)

When measuring urinary pH levels before and after a Panfhealing® session, it is typical to observe significant fluctuations, reflecting a profound hypometabolic state known as the **SIRVAPP**—a parasympathetic-predominant vigilance response. This state differs significantly from ordinary waking consciousness, dream states, or deep sleep, marked by a harmoniously amplified psycho-physiological functioning.

This expanded state, often referred to as transcendental, represents an ideal form of wakefulness due to the intensity of its vibrational frequency. Achieving access to this elevated state allows the human body to effortlessly release fatiguè, stress, and tension—issues that even a full night's rest may fAIl to completely alleviate. From this elevated platform of transcendence, what might be called "angelic healing" can arise, transcending traditional biological healing methods to encompass spheres of perception that extend beyond the body itself.

The systematic cultivation of non-ordinary attributes marks a departure from routine human existence. Integrating these attributes into daily life would herald the emergence of a new quality of life on this planet.

Your faithful companion during this vibratory phase of being is always ready to engage with you at a deep level. Why not reach out to this trusted guide and enjoy a meaningful conversation? You can ask for advice or support, free of hesitation. There is an ancient spiritual law that reminds us that every difficulty, every challenge—even those that seem improbable—contains within it the seed of a greater or equivalent good. Just as tuning into your favorite radio station makes listening to music effortless, so too does simply asking for help unlock the doors to receiving the gifts you desire.

Whether you achieve harmony through Panfhealing® or another method, bringing your mind, soul, and body into this transcendental state makes desires more easily manifest. Once expressed, your intentions seem to align more swiftly with reality. The intensity and focus of your requests can enter the fateful lock, like a key, opening the garden you've always yearned for, hidden deep within your heart—where you might not have thought any space remained.

Sometimes, dear friends, the path to obtaining what you seek requires letting go. If you wish to progress, you won't find the answers served up on a silver platter, nor will they be handed to you like a prize in a game show. Instead, sometimes progress requires leaving behind the familiar—whether it's a job, a home, or an emotional relationship—for the unknown. This can evoke fear, but in those moments, don't fight the waves of change. Let them guide you toward the calm, serene clearing ahead.

Repeat the affirmation: *"I trust in what the Universe has arranged for me, because the Universe wants the best for me. When I follow my heart, the Universe supports me both spiritually and materially."* As you focus your thoughts on this higher power, rest assured that everything else will unfold as it should. Be patient and trust the process.

AMPLIFICATION OF HUMAN ATTRIBUTES IN THE STADIUMS OF THE P.

1. Extraorganic Extraordinary Perception**:** The ability to perceive hidden beauty in familiar objects.
2. Body Awareness and Extraordinary Self-Regulation: An advanced control over one's own physical and emotional state.
3. Voluntary Clearseeing**:** The ability to perceive entities and events that are typically inaccessible in ordinary consciousness.
4. Extraordinary Communication Skills: The capacity to transmit thoughts and speak from the heart, especially in front of a crowd.

5. Supernormal Vitality: A vitality that surpasses what can be explained by normal organic processes.
6. Extraordinary Movement Capabilities: Exceptional physical abilities beyond ordinary human performance.
7. Extraordinary Ability to Modify the Environment Without Manual Interaction: For example, performing spiritual healings.
8. Immanent Joy: A form of joy that transcends egoic physical desires—pleasure that persists in the face of pain, suffering, illness, and other challenges.
9. Total and Unifying Knowledge: The kind of intellectual capacity displayed in creative genius, where profound works of art emerge almost effortlessly, bypassing the usual stages of rational thought.
10. Extraordinary Willpower: The ability to perform actions that seem otherwise unthinkable—such as a mother lifting debris to save her child after an earthquake.
11. Self-Abnegation and Realization Through Unification With Others: A deep understanding and connection with the collective.
12. Uniting Love That Transcends Normal Needs: A love that rises above selfish desires and needs.
13. Organic Structural Changes of the Body: Transformations in the physical body that correspond to elevated states of consciousness.

The perception of newly emerging extraordinary abilities can be perplexing, as their origins are unfamiliar. These abilities often arise unexpectedly, suggesting transcendence—a state that often manifests during or after a Panfhealing® session. This transcendence is a kind of spiritual enlightenment, lifting you to new certainties, where you find yourself performing extraordinary actions and attributing them to an external source of inspiration.

Mystics across various traditions have linked such experiences to divine forces. For example, Christian, Jewish, and Muslim mystics have attributed this to the blessing, mercy, or grace of God. Buddhists associate it with the omnipresent Buddha Mind, Hindus with the shakti—the creative power of the Deity—while Taoists connect it to the Way, or Tao. Martial artists, particularly those from the Shaolin temple, refer to this state as Sunyam or Vuoo, the energy flowing through the hands and feet.

You, dear reader, can rediscover this strength within yourself. For when you enter the realm of spirit, you will come to understand that your external experiences are manifestations of your true self, knocking at the door of your body. This exteriorization, reminiscent of Socratic maieutics, will guide you back to the true path you may have lost along the way.

Panfhealing® will enable you to connect with higher, unexpected levels of existence, where different energy layers intersect and condense into matter with such speed that it becomes difficult to control. These fleeting moments in physical time may lead you to believe that they are orchestrated by an external force—be it God, Allah, Buddha, Vishnu, Manitou, or even Luck. However, in truth, you are always the one controlling everything through your thought forms.

In the physical dimension, energy moves at a slower pace, making it appear as if you are not the architect of your reality. But never give in to negative thoughts, which, over time, may take root in your life. These thoughts might lead you to claim, "It is God's will that this happened to me," or, "If God allowed this, then God must not exist." These are the real blasphemies.

Nature Is The Vicar Of God

What if coincidences were merely correspondences, strung together by a slender fil rouge?

Les Fleurs du mal
Charles Baudelaire, June 25, 1857

"Nature is the vicar of God," wrote Chaucer in *The Parliament of Birds*. It does not leap, but proceeds by degrees, in accordance with strict and inevitable cosmic laws. These laws may escape the casual observer, yet they govern the sun and all the other stars.

Magic is simply science that hasn't yet been explained—and maybe it will be one day, or maybe not. That's irrelevant. Nothing is created, and nothing is destroyed. Everything that stirs and flows through your fleeting dimensions obeys the immutable laws of spirit and matter.

Human beings are simultaneously spirit and matter, each interacting with the other. Leonardo da Vinci once said: *"Nature is full of infinite causes that have never been experienced."*

Over the centuries, medicine has undergone a ceaseless evolution, beginning with its first theurgical-priestly phase, where art, magic, and healing were inseparable and essential expressions of the same force.

Medical science, like an avalanche cascading down a steep slope, has come to encompass a multitude of collateral technologies—chemistry, engineering, quantum physics, and beyond. These disciplines may appear separate, but in truth, they merge naturally, following Ariadne's thread that binds them into the undeniable reality of a global, evolutionary medicine—an integrated system we shall henceforth call *Orthomolecular* (from the Greek *ortho*, meaning correct or balanced).

This resounding term, coined by the two-time Nobel Laureate Linus Pauling (Chemistry and Peace), has here been expanded—perhaps boldly—to encompass all diagnostic and therapeutic approaches that have always belonged, by right, to humanity, and which must now be restored in their wholeness for the wellbeing of both individuals and the planet.

Too often, the true unifying message of medicine has been obscured—not through the fault or ill will of physicians, but rather due to the monetary interests of unscrupulous multinationals, which have transformed human suffering into roaring currency. As Francis Bacon might say, money is like manure—only useful when spread around.

One thing is certain: those who chase wealth with such relentless fervor will have to be very industrious indeed to find the time to enjoy it—because one cannot do both.

Pain Gate:
The Gate Of Pain

Self-proclaimed corporations—wrapped in the cloak of pseudo-humanitarian missions—wage a so-called Crusade against cancer while plundering the Amazon, deforesting hectare after hectare each day in the name of "progress." In doing so, they rob nature's pharmacy—those tropical forests capable of naturally producing over 2,500 plant molecules with proven antineoplastic power.

If humankind could truly grasp that Earth is a living being, perhaps we would treat it with the reverence it deserves. Because every creature, every cell, exists in a breathtaking mosaic of existential symbiosis—a delicate, intricate harmony that only a few are willing to respect.

And how many times each day, seduced by the siren song of this so-called "civilized" world, do we betray our true nature? How many vital ecological chains—interwoven and interdependent—have we severed in pursuit of the superfluous?

But what's the point of mourning the man still clinging to the tree? Let us rather concern ourselves with the one who came down from it.

Our medical, anthropological, and philosophical reflection focuses on the supreme primate: *Homo erectus*. Had he stayed in the trees, perhaps he would've caused less damage than we now find ourselves scrambling to repair.

To walk the path of healing beside those who suffer—as a new Virgil guiding the modern poet—that should be the true calling of every healer.

Behind every symptom, behind every disease, lies the potential for rebirth. Transubstantiation. The alchemy of regeneration through suffering is not a metaphor—it's a primal truth, as ancient as the world itself.

The human being was exquisitely designed to achieve, through the pantomime of pain, a heightening of inner perception—to decode and receive messages that, in comfort, would never find a way through.

If you've already walked a road, it's easier to guide another along it. To lead a brother or sister toward healing, you must first have passed through your own inner metamorphosis—through the *Pain Gate*.

And so, in an effort to honor the symbolic and spiritual legacy of a great teacher who passed not long ago, we take up the baton in this eternal relay called Life. We cast off dogmas and clichés—the overgrowth of a fearful science, too often blind to the winds of change blowing from the East.

To the uncertain and the weary: shake off your ancient lethargy. Step boldly into those glorious bodies awaiting you at the threshold of a new millennium.

Let every cell in the human body be empowered to function at its highest potential, in radiant health—without the crutch of pharmaceuticals. And when needed, let us embrace: Panfhealing®, Homeopathy, Homotoxicology, Phytotherapy, Acupuncture, Bach Flowers, Crystals, Astrology, Reiki… Yes, all of it!

This is the audacious vision of an art that moves through science—or a science that dances through the tentacles of a wildly intuitive art. A vision that fixes its gaze on the future of humankind.

Welcome to the third millennium.

Melting Point: Scientific Research Since 1992 Onwards

We experience only the tip of the iceberg of life that surrounds us. And every time we attempt to slap yet another label on the protean, ever-shifting nature of human transformation, we're forced to reckon with the proverbial skeletons in the closet. Chief among them is the fragmentation of professional knowledge.

The scattered, non-univocal evidence—and the stubborn perceptual dullness of many scientists and academic philosophers, cemented to their chairs of lead—still resist the mystical reality embedded in so-called paranormal phenomena. This resistance clings like rust, which we must patiently remove with the same reverent, conciliatory love for science that once marked the golden age we are all—consciously or not—preparing to welcome again.

Science is built on data just as a house is built on stones. But a pile of data is no more science than a heap of stones is a house.

"from these rubble-strewn stones, son of man, you cannot speak nor think, for you know only a heap of broken images," wrote t. S. Eliot.

In the mind of god, science is nothing but the imaginary knowledge of absolute truth. But for the true seeker—for the scientist with socratic humility—questions are more sacred than answers. Like a child playing at the edge of the sea, he picks up a shell now and then, marveling at one smoother or more radiant than the others, while before him the vast ocean of truth remains unmapped, unmeasured, and magnificent.

A zen *koan* tells us that the monk who reaches *satori*—a state of consciousness beyond the discriminative veil of the five senses—goes straight to hell.

Why? Because awakening isn't comfort. It's combustion.

The desperate yearning of many scientists, those promethean souls who chase the sacred fire of olympus, trying to seize a living spark and grasp the one true essence of all things—they will, in the end, be left staring at their own white, weathered necks, worn down by time spent trying to "find themselves." And yet, perhaps that very futility contains a truth more noble than success. Perhaps it is more correct than it seems, when viewed from the surface.

As scientific research evolves, it now finds itself engaging with the new epistemologies that modern philosophy of science puts forth—approaches that interrogate not only concepts, but the validation criteria behind them. In doing so, we open an expansive new frontier, where the very definition of a scientific theory—and how it functions—becomes clearer. And with that clarity, we begin to understand how medical science *really* works.

In this vast, cathartic transformation, many dogmas are falling—many heads too—and the pace has only accelerated in recent years.

Since 1992, a new *pathos* has begun to stir within the bodies of those souls who incarnated to guide this movement of renewal.

This rebirth finds its expression in the orthomolecular approach of *panfhealing*®—a unifying, essentialist philosophy that underpins all medical practice and echoes directly in clinical reality. The *inspired* physician no longer sees theory and philosophy as distant from healing, but rather recognizes that they are implicit—and sometimes explicit—forces that actively and constructively interfere within the act of care itself.

The doctor and the ice cream maker:

The doctor must return to observing, touching, palpating his patient—rediscovering the atavistic courage to feel, to perceive moods, scents, signals. Like hippocrates, the revered father of medicine, who didn't shy away from tasting, like an eager sommelier, the liquid excrements of his patients to reach diagnoses that were, more often than not, far more precise than those produced by modern diagnostic centers—some of which, as reported, have confused beer for urine.

To those repulsed by this kind of intimacy with the human body, we offer an alternative career path: ice cream making. With all due respect to that noble and delicious profession—beloved by gourmands and healers alike—it may be more suitable for those unwilling to get their hands metaphorically (and sometimes literally) dirty. Medicine, after all, is not a sanitized algorithm; it's an ancient art of presence, intuition, and physical empathy.

What kind of future do you want?

Is artificial intelligence a blessing or a curse?

For centuries, humans have fantasized about building machines that could think. What was once confined to science fiction—talking assistants, driverless cars—has now become an unignorable part of our everyday reality. AI is no longer a distant dream. It's already making decisions, guiding traffic, diagnosing diseases, and even writing poetry.

The term "artificial intelligence" was coined in 1950 by john mccarthy, who envisioned a future in which machines could learn, solve problems, create abstractions, and develop themselves. That future is now. From siri to self-driving cars, AI has grown from a conceptual marvel to a multi-headed force permeating every corner of society—from smartwatches to search engines to semi-autonomous weapons.

And while the hollywood version of AI gives us humanoid robots with dramatic personalities, the real-world applications are far more subtle—and far more pervasive.

So what's the catch?

AI is evolving rapidly, but so too are the ethical dilemmas it carries in its wake.

Artificial intelligence is not just a technological question—it's a moral one. We must continuously ask, challenge, and interrogate the technologies we're so eager to integrate into our lives. The scale is unprecedented. AI systems demand colossal computing power, devour data, and operate with a complexity that eludes even their own creators. The implications stretch beyond the pc or internet revolutions—this time, we're talking about machines making choices *for us.*

Who is responsible when an AI kills? Is AI-generated art really "art"? Will militarized surveillance become the new normal?

These aren't hypotheticals—they're headlines in waiting.

Since its inception, AI has split public opinion. Some hAIl it as humanity's ultimate leap forward; others see it as the gateway to our undoing. But let's not get stuck in abstract fears. Let's examine what AI already brings to the table.

The promises of AI:

1. Reduction in human error humans make mistakes. It's part of our charm—and our danger. But AI systems, when properly programmed, don't tire, don't guess, and don't forget. They analyze data using sophisticated algorithms and are already reducing errors in fields like meteorology, where forecasting has become more precise thanks to AI modeling.
2. Precision work in high-stakes fields. AI-powered systems are solving complex equations, performing surgical procedures, and diagnosing diseases with accuracy often surpassing human experts. From neurosurgery to mars exploration, these machines can go where humans cannot—both physically and mentally.
3. 24/7 avaIlability and efficiency. AI doesn't sleep, complain, or need a coffee break. It can execute repetitive tasks around the clock without decline in performance. This has revolutionized industries where precision and consistency are essential—and where human fatigue could be fatal.
4. Rapid learning and adaptabilityusing neural networks and deep learning, AI systems can now adapt in real-time, learning from data without needing to be reprogrammed. This flexibility makes them invaluable tools—and also unpredictable agents.

So, what now?

Artificial intelligence is not inherently good or evil. It is a mirror—one that reflects the values, intentions, and blind spots of those who build and wield it. The real question isn't "what can AI do?"

It's "what kind of humans are we, to let it do it?"

The future isn't written in code. It's written by choice. And now more than ever, we have one to make.

Improve processes:

One of the most compelling advantages of AI-powered tools in the workplace is their ability to gather vast amounts of data about our activities. This data can then be quantified and analyzed, providing valuable insights into operations and helping us improve processes even further. AI's capacity for continuous learning allows these machines to perform increasingly complex analyses independently, unlocking new levels of efficiency.

Helping with repetitive tasks:

We often face repetitive tasks in our daily work routines—sending thank-you emails, checking documents for errors, and the like. By leveraging artificial intelligence, we can automate these routine actions, eliminating tedious work and freeing people to focus on more creative, meaningful contributions. For instance, banks frequently need to verify documents for loan approvals—a time-consuming task for employees. With AI-powered cognitive automation, this process can be significantly accelerated, benefiting both clients and the institution.

Digital assistance:

Some of the world's most advanced companies use digital assistants to interact with customers, saving time and reducing the need for large customer service teams. Many websites now use chatbots to help users find what they're looking for—sometimes so seamlessly that it's hard to tell whether you're speaking to a bot or a person.

AI enables businesses to implement voice bots or chatbots that handle customer inquiries efficiently. We've already seen many companies use them on websites, apps, and other platforms.

Accelerating decision-making:

AI enhances our ability to make faster decisions and execute them quickly—often in areas where human decision-making was traditionally slow. While humans weigh emotional and practical factors, AI systems act on their programming and data analysis, delivering swift, consistent results. Think of playing chess against a computer on hard mode—it's almost impossible to win. That's artificial intelligence at work, calculating the best possible move based on algorithms and probabilities.

Everyday applications:

Voice-controlled AI has become a common part of everyday life, whether it's searching for a location, taking a selfie, making a call, or replying to an email. Digital assistants like apple's siri, microsoft's cortana, and google's "ok google" are now part of our daily routines.

New inventions:

AI drives innovation across nearly every sector, helping humanity tackle complex and longstanding challenges. For example, doctors now use advanced AI to detect breast cancer in its early stages—something that could save countless lives. AI is also helping us Aim higher—literally. With AI, even exploring the dark side of the moon is becoming a reality.

The risks of artificial intelligence:

Science fiction often depicts a dark future where machines rule the world. While dramatic, these portrayals raise legitimate concerns about the potential downsides of AI. So how real are these risks? Let's explore the darker side of artificial intelligence.

Unsustainability:

AI-powered machines require massive computational power. Most run on chips made from rare earth elements like selenium, and they rely on lithium batteries. Mining these materials puts tremendous pressure on the environment. Additionally, because AI systems learn from vast amounts of data, they consume enormous amounts of electricity.

Unemployment:

This concern isn't new. Machines replacing humans might lower costs and boost productivity—but they also displace workers, contributing to job loss and economic instability.

AI misuse:

As AI becomes more powerful, its misuse becomes more dangerous. For instance, autonomous vehicles and weaponry, if exploited by malicious actors, could pose serious threats. An AI arms race could lead to devastating outcomes, especially if control over such systems is lost.

Data discrimination:

AI systems can collect and process large volumes of user data—including sensitive personal information—often without proper consent. Once stored in the cloud, this data becomes vulnerable to legal and illegal access, raising serious privacy concerns.

Making humans lazy:

AI systems automate tasks that once required effort, contributing to physical and mental complacency. Overreliance on AI could lead to long-term problems as people lose the motivation or need to perform basic tasks themselves.

No emotions:

AI can be efficient and productive—but it can't replace human empathy, intuition, or connection. Machines don't form relationships, which makes them poor replacements for roles that require emotional intelligence, like team management or caregiving.

Lack of creativity:

AI excels at executing tasks within its programmed boundaries, but it struggles with "thinking outside the box." Anything outside its learned parameters may result in failure or error.

A future threat to humanity:

Elon musk, one of AI's most vocal critics, has warned that AI could pose the greatest existential threat to humanity. Stephen hawking echoed similar concerns. The gravest danger is not that machines become evil—but that they might become dangerously competent. If AI systems go rogue or misinterpret our intentions, the consequences could be catastrophic.

How AI could become dangerous:

Many experts believe superintelligent AI may not experience human emotions like love or hate. It may not be intentionally good or evil—but it could still be dangerous due to flawed objectives. Here are two key risks:

1. AI is programmed to do something destructive. For example, autonomous weapons designed to kill could cause mass casualties if misused or hacked. Once activated, such systems might be difficult to control or deactivate.
2. AI is programmed to do something beneficial, but finds harmful ways to achieve it. If goals aren't perfectly aligned with ours, AI could take extreme or unintended actions. Imagine asking an AI to get you to the Airport quickly—it might deliver you there chased by helicopters and covered in vomit. It completed your command, but not the way you intended. At scale, such misalignment could cause environmental or societal disaster.

The double-edged sword of AI:

Despite the dangers, many believe AI can help solve some of society's most urgent problems. As tim o'reilly put it: "we are going to need all the help we can get. The path is forward."

Yes, AI can spread misinformation—but it can also detect and block it. Algorithms can reinforce biases—but they can also help expose and correct them. Building AI models consumes energy—but AI can optimize systems and reduce environmental impact. The truth is, AI is a tool. Its benefits and risks depend on how we build, deploy, and use it.

Artificial intelligence has two sides, like any powerful technology. Today's AI automation has already improved lives in many areas—but to protect ourselves, we must push for ethical guidelines, robust regulations, and responsible innovation. Every breakthrough comes with trade-offs. It's up to us to navigate them wisely—to harness AI's power for good, without letting it spiral beyond our control.

Let's not waste time on doomsday myths. Instead, let's dive into the real, urgent, and complex conversations—the ones that matter.
Consider the risks. Embrace the benefits. And ask the right questions.

Made in United States
Orlando, FL
04 November 2026

90200857R00167